STEP-TRAINING
WORKOUT

QUICK AND EFFECTIVE WORKOUTS FOR THE WHOLE BODY

SOFIA
SJÖSTRÖM STÅHL

PHOTOGRAPHY BY ERIK DELEXIT
TRANSLATED BY GUN PENHOAT

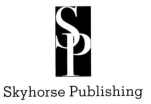

Skyhorse Publishing

For Kim—because you make me believe I can

Text © Sofia Sjöström Ståhl, 2016, 2019.
Photography © Erik Dilexit, 2016, 2019.
First published by Fitnessförlaget in Stockholm, Sweden in 2016 as *Trappträning*.
First Skyhorse Publishing edition, 2019.

Skyhorse Publishing books may be purchased in bulk at special discounts for sales promotion, corporate gifts, fund-raising, or educational purposes. Special editions can also be created to specifications. For details, contact the Special Sales Department, Skyhorse Publishing, 307 West 36th Street, 11th Floor, New York, NY 10018 or info@skyhorsepublishing.com.

Skyhorse® and Skyhorse Publishing® are registered trademarks of Skyhorse Publishing, Inc.®, a Delaware corporation. Visit our website at www.skyhorsepublishing.com.

10 9 8 7 6 5 4 3 2 1

Library of Congress Cataloging-in-Publication Data is available on file.

Book design by Anders Timrén

Print ISBN: 978-1-5107-3019-9
Ebook ISBN: 978-1-5107-3024-3

Printed in China

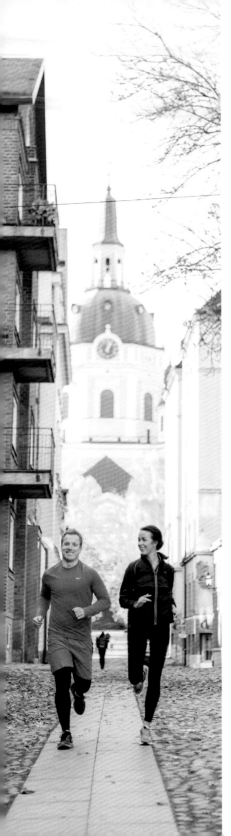

CONTENTS

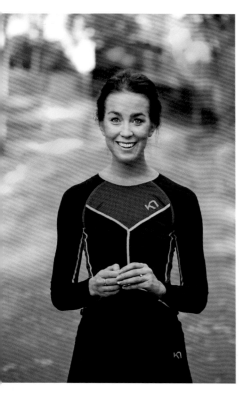

INTRODUCTION

My relationship with exercise has never been very consistent—we have had our ups and downs over the years. Physical training was an integral part of my life growing up; I competed in cross-country skiing, which meant that I did several workouts a week and went to long training camps in both summer and winter. Aside from all the hours on the ski trails, I also participated in off-season training and triathlons, and have covered many miles on roller-skis. In addition, I spent much of my free time at the stables and rode horses for over a decade. I've also run cross-country and have tried out most team sports and several para-sports during my years as a personal assistant. You get the picture: I'm quite the jock.

Exercise and physical activities have, quite simply, always taken up a lot of my and my family's spare time. This changed somewhat when, upon graduation, I moved to the United States, and then to Oslo, Norway. There, partying and having fun were far more tempting than putting myself through sweaty workouts. Later, when I moved back to Stockholm, Sweden, and got my credentials to become a personal trainer, I found my way back to my old routines, and my schedule filled up with exercise. I discovered strength training; I started rising early in the morning to crawl around outside doing military boot-camp workouts. Then everything changed when I became ill, suffering from burnout and depression.

My body became incredibly weak and I didn't train for a hundred days. I neither wanted to nor was able to engage in exercise. I fought hard to regain some motivation to get myself going again, but often found myself unable to rally. Who was I without my training? Once I began moving again and really rediscovered the joys of exercising, things almost immediately went off the rails again. I damaged my elbows so severely during a workout that I almost tore my muscles. Nearly two years of intense physical therapy sapped all my energy, and I had to start back at square one.

What I'm trying to tell you, by recounting this long tale of woe, is that I was the girl bursting with energy, who had training deeply embedded in her DNA. You know, the one who was exhilarated at the prospect of going out into the woods and running until she came close to throwing up. I loved to sweat and to feel the taste of blood on my tongue. But I have had to face the harsh realities of being a jock. I've had days when I physically could not do a thing because my body was too exhausted to move; I've injured myself to the point where I was unable to lift so much as pitcher of water; and I've gone all the way to the gym, only to realize that I should not be there, and gone back home to lie on the couch again. I do understand that working out can spark some of the most fantastic feelings ever, but also the most horrible pain. I also get that people who are wholly committed to training can often be incredibly challenging to be around.

However, I've always appreciated what is simple as well as effective. That is probably why I always go back to step training. There are stretches of time when I don't do any step training, but then I find myself back at the foot of a flight of stairs again, ready to take on the challenge once more. What gives me the biggest rush? To be out on a walk and to suddenly feel the urge to run a few intervals on the stairs. It's so darn simple, after all!

That's why I wanted to write a book about exercise that wasn't intimidating; I wanted it to be welcoming and to include something for everyone. This book is for anyone who already enjoys training, as well as for whoever has not quite made it out of the starting blocks yet. This book can be used by those who train to build functional strength, as well as by those who are looking for a reliable workout to provide their body with the basics. In short, it is for anyone seeking an effective—and easy-to-follow—training plan.

You can use this book no matter your relationship to exercise and regardless of where you find yourself along the fitness spectrum. There's always a set of stairs somewhere, waiting to be pressed into service. If you're a complete newbie, start out by simply walking up and down a few flights. Take one step at a time and you will reach the top. Keep in mind that things don't need to get any more intricate than this.

With warm greetings! *Sofia*

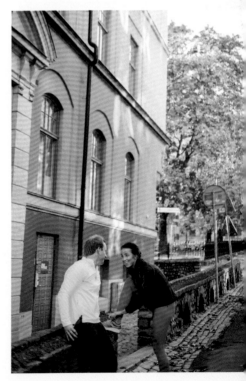

WHY STEP TRAINING?

I think it's a pity that we make everything so complicated these days. The best we can do for ourselves is to move our bodies, and the dumbest thing we can do is to make this movement convoluted. That's why I'd like to introduce you to something so simple that it might be considered unacceptable: step training. What? Real training done on stairs? That's right. I began using stairs to exercise a long time ago, in an attempt to find new ways to challenge my body. You might think that climbing stairs as fast as possible is all there is to it, and then it's done. Trust me—that's not all; there are so many other things you can do!

Simple training is my thing. You know, exercise that's fun and straightforward; where you can just lace up your shoes and get going. That's what I feel step training is all about. The equipment can be found just about anywhere, and it's free and accessible to everyone. I love using the stairs that are located about a hundred yards from my home, which are completely covered in greenery in summertime. I'll go there when I don't feel like moving, and I become motivated again. I'll go there when I need to vent my frustrations. I'll go there when I want to train to the point of exhaustion, and when I want to challenge my body in different ways. It's so easy to provide your body with much-needed movement using a flight of stairs. Have you ever thought about it? If not, no matter. Hopefully, your curiosity will now have been aroused, and you'll be tempted to make your way to the nearest set of stairs to try out an exercise or two.

There several advantages to performing a few of your workouts on stairs: you'll see many exercises with fresh eyes, you'll discover the importance of finding your center of gravity, and you'll realize that balance and coordination are heavily involved. You'll see results.

In this book, I've chosen to focus on training that challenges your strength, balance, coordination, fitness, and mobility. As an added bonus, you'll even get to experience that great, slightly devil-may-care feeling of not giving a second thought to what people say or think while you're out doing fun exercises on stairs. I believe we also become mentally stronger by putting ourselves into these types of situations from time to time.

Each section of this book (strength, fitness, and balance) contains a few basic exercises that each have three variations. These variations are there to stimulate your imagination, to work different parts of your body, and to raise the effort required to complete the exercise. And since I love to talk about training (I consider it to be an integral part of health), with an emphasis on the body as a whole, I couldn't resist adding a few thoughts on the subject on page 89. Think of them as words to guide you down the road toward a more balanced view of exercise, health, and, who knows, maybe even a different outlook on life itself.

WHAT IS ENOUGH FOR YOU

In my opinion, good health means that there is balance (or perhaps more accurately, a search for balance) between the different areas that make up our lives. To create a sense of well-being, we must strive to make time for work, rest, exercise, movement, our social life, quiet time, eating, stress, demands, as well as recovery. We do stray from this goal from time to time, when we push ourselves intensely for a few weeks, but we need to know that this period is finite and that afterward we need time for recuperation. Only then can we achieve balance.

I don't always need my movements to feel like formal exercise in order to appreciate them. What's most important is that I move my body. In my mind, exercise is that half hour spent cycling into town, or playing a game of badminton on the lawn outside the summerhouse, or deciding to learn handstands (why not?) and practicing them tirelessly. It might be jumping on the trampoline with my nieces and nephews or going for a long ramble in the woods. It can mean walking to a stairway and sprinting up the steps a few times or stretching out on a Pilates ball in front of the computer to take a break during the workday. I strongly believe that we must begin to value all of our movements, be they part of active play or physical training, in order to find that magical state of equilibrium. Everyday movements, in combination with efficient training, give rise to something very good, namely health. That's why we need both types of motion.

So how do we go about doing this training—the integral part of our lives where many of us get stuck when we wish to boost our health? Nowadays there is a tendency to make exercise unconventional and elaborate. It often turns into a complicated project, if not a form of punishment, instead of being an activity that improves and strengthens us step by step. I had the advantage of practically growing up on cross-country ski trails and participating in rigorous workouts as well as outdoor spontaneous play, which for me has made training and movement natural parts of my life. I need to stretch my legs, to move my body, and to breathe fresh air every day to feel good. Over the years, my greatest luxury is having learned to value simple movement as highly as my workouts. This means that my days turn out fine even when planned exercise sessions don't fit into my schedule, because I'll make a point of walking to the office or doing a headstand in front of the TV at night. Using your body doesn't always require thinking ahead or learning new moves. What do you consider to be training?

I suggest that you keep your feet firmly planted on the ground when you plan your workouts. Most of us are ordinary (and commendable) garden-variety exercisers who train just to improve our well-being, yet it's so easy to be lured in by routines that seem geared toward the exercise elite. Even the average "Joe" or "Jane" who works full-time and has a family and a social life needs to train in an efficient way that lets him or her get more out of their everyday existence. The kindest gift we can give ourselves is simple, effective, and, at times, tough workouts that challenge and strengthen both our body and mind. If you do a few hardcore training sessions per week, you'll be fine just doing some complementary activity like walking, doing handstands, or spontaneous play on other days of the week.

Of course, my recommendation is that you perform some of your workouts on the nearest set of stairs, but no matter what type of training you choose, remember to appreciate the smallest of movements. Even the short, five-minute sessions featured in this book will contribute to your good health.

Don't complicate things. Let the simple pleasure of being active be your guide.

TRAIN LESS OFTEN, BUT BETTER

These days, it's very easy to be tricked into thinking that we need to do as much as possible and train excessively for our efforts to even make a dent. It's not uncommon for many people to become stressed out by goals that are set too high as they train relentlessly over the first few weeks after summer vacation. I believe you should do the opposite. As I hear from more and more people who are despondent because they can't find the time to do it all, I've become convinced that we need to break away from the tenet that more is always better.

I want to try to make you understand that it is not the amount of training that counts, it's what you do and how you do it. You will probably feel better if you choose a few moments during the week when you can concentrate on yourself and your training—and let yourself be happy and satisfied with this—rather than to trying to shoehorn an exercise session in every other day. We reap the most benefits when we set realistic and reasonable goals and consider anything above and beyond a bonus.

You may be familiar with the feeling of planning out several training sessions throughout the week, only to have the days go by and to realize you simply don't have the time to tackle them all. Disappointment is a fact; you feel regret over what you did not accomplish, instead of appreciating what you were actually able to do. It doesn't matter how good the workout was or how much fun it turned out to be, you still only focus on what you missed. I encourage you to lower the bar a little, and to practice always giving yourself a pat on the back for what you have achieved, instead of beating yourself up over what you didn't do. Plan on a few training sessions per week and think of whatever else you can add to that as a nice perk.

Get it right by making your preplanned exercise sessions truly your time. Turn off the phone, dare not to be social, and focus on yourself while you're training. This will improve the quality of your workouts and your sense of satisfaction, leading you to see positive results.

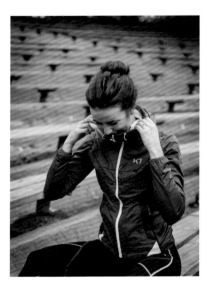

"Turn off the phone, dare not to be social, and focus on yourself while you're training."

THE BENEFITS OF THIS TYPE OF TRAINING

There are many benefits to step training. Here are eight reasons why I love step training (and soon you will too!)

- **Positive results.** The workouts are effective. Many will notice quick results, because the exercises are done on different ground levels and emphasize different centers of gravity, which makes them more challenging.

- **You'll get outside.** Today it is widely accepted—proven, even—that time spent outside enhances our well-being. Many believe that time spent in the fresh air makes them feel more alert, helps them de-stress, and clears up brain fog. Training outside is almost addictive, as the endorphins from training and the air in our lungs go together so well.

- **You move at different levels.** Modern-day human beings rarely come in contact with different ground levels. We have smooth, asphalt-covered roads; effort-saving planning designs; and many other conveniences. Many become stuck in a training rut and few put their body through unfamiliar movements. By training on steps, you're forced to meet the challenge of really lifting your feet, of trying new angles, and of coping with a shifting center of gravity. It's excellent for maintaining—or developing—a functionally strong body.

"You can take familiar exercises and freshen them up and make them more challenging by doing them on the stairs."

- **It's free.** There are stairs almost everywhere (if there are no stairs, there will be a slope). The exercises are free and accessible, and the necessary equipment is available to anyone, in order to develop strength, fitness, balance, and coordination.

- **It's flexible.** You decide what level to use for your training. You can perform basic exercises and start out by walking briskly up and down the stairs to raise your heart rate. You can take familiar exercises and freshen them up, making them more challenging by doing them on the stairs.

- **It's easy to make progress.** With the inherently brilliant design of stairs, and a bit of imagination, you can easily increase the difficulty and weight load of your workouts.

- **It can be a social occasion, if you'd like it to be.** Stairs make room for more than one person at a time, so if you enjoy company while you train, you can ask someone to work out with you. It's more energizing and often more enjoyable.

- **You get to go to a new "gym" each time.** You can bring this book and its exercises with you when you're on vacation, if you travel for work, and whenever you want a change of scenery. There are stairs of all types and in places all over the world. Maybe you can create a new game out of finding the best set of steps during your next vacation time.

GET RESULTS

When you first add step training to your routine, it might be a good idea to focus on building a strong foundation. Don't get carried away thinking you can immediately proceed to the hardest exercises five days a week. Give your body a chance to get to that point in a realistic time frame, which will lessen your risk of getting injured. There's no rush. To see results, you must train regularly, listen to your body, and dare to challenge yourself at even intervals. Don't underestimate the importance of balance and movement—they'll help you build that sturdy base you'll need to tackle the harder workouts.

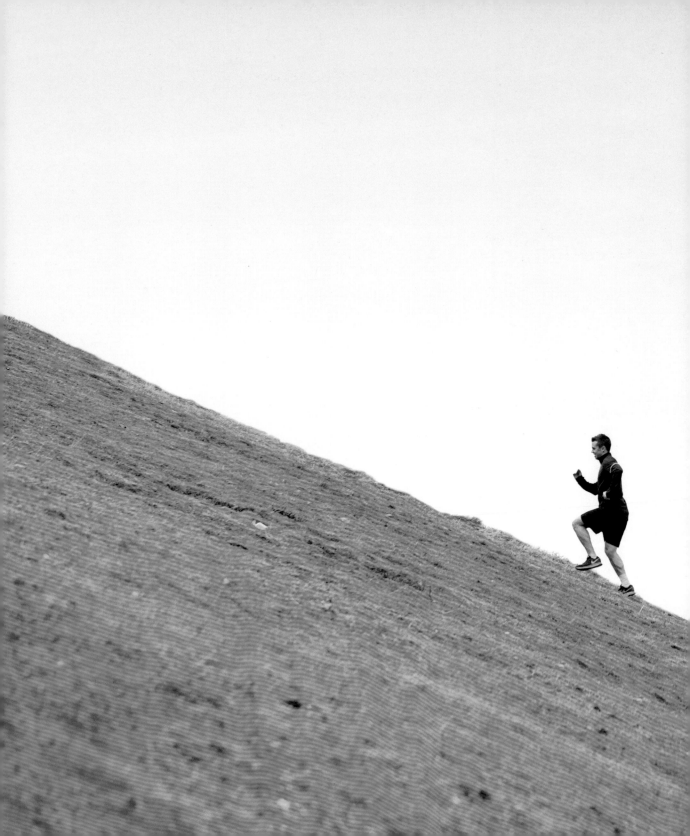

TRAINING ON A SLOPE

Many of these exercises can also be done on a slope, if you don't feel comfortable starting off right away on stairs or if you do not have access to steps. There are many advantages to working out on a slope from time to time. Among other things, you get to try out different surfaces and run on hilly terrain. Your cardio fitness will be tested. You can make the intervals longer or find a steeper incline. It's important that you modify each exercise if you choose to use a slope instead of the stairs. Try out the exercises. You might need to adjust your center of gravity a little to perform them correctly, or maybe run a little longer during the intervals to become winded. Another good practice is to combine a few step exercises with interval training on a steep slope, so don't let one site rule out another when finding places to train. This book's aim is really just to make you think outside the box and seek new ways to move your body, so be creative!

HOW TO USE THIS BOOK

It's essential that you be honest with yourself if you want to get the most out of your training, and that you don't begin with the most challenging exercises right off the bat. After reading this book, I suggest you find the nearest set of stairs that look promising and start getting acquainted with them. Perhaps you'll finish your next walk or jog with a few quick sprints up the steps just to get a feel for them, or you might even go straight for some of this book's exercises.

It's important to be familiar with the different levels when you train on steps so that you don't injure yourself and so your sense of balance is tested. Keep in mind that you might need to begin with the basic exercises before trying any variations. Always be aware of where you place your feet and stay close to a handrail so you can hold on to it if you need to.

It's not my intention to have you perform all the exercises and programs in your first week. It's a good idea to start out with two or three basic moves to familiarize yourself with the exercise equipment (refer to the basic program suggestion at the bottom of the page), especially if you have never trained on stairs before. If you wish to challenge yourself significantly during the upcoming weeks, you can incorporate any of the book's training plans (starting on page 84) into your own current training schedule.

BASIC PROGRAM

TIME: 15 minutes
BASIC EXERCISES: Bear Crawl, Stair Jump, and Balance with Leg Lift
WARM-UP: Mountain Climbers

HOW TO: Warm up by doing Mountain Climbers in intervals (10 seconds active, 10 seconds rest x 8). Then perform one exercise at a time, for 1 minute each. Repeat the exercises in 3 circuits. Rest for 30 to 45 seconds between each circuit.

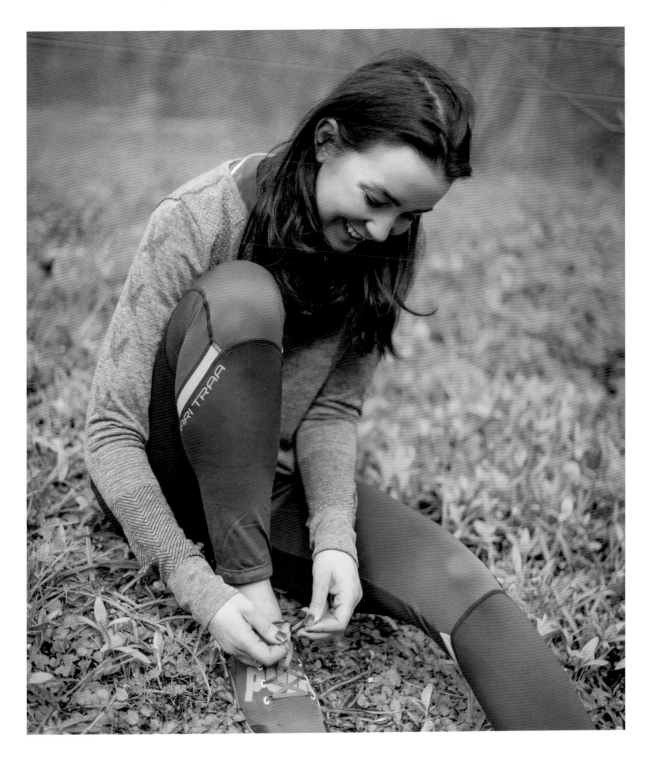

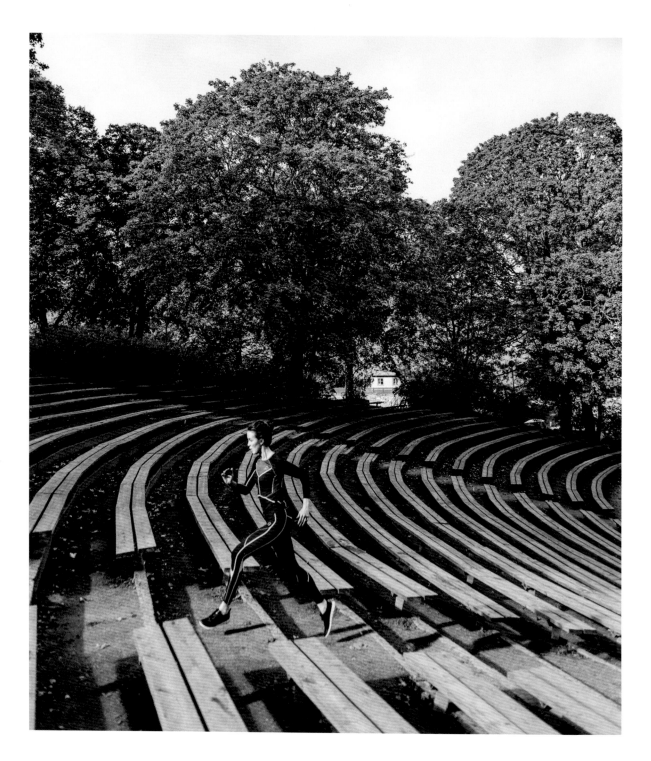

THE EXERCISES

We've come to the section that explains all the exercises. I have split them into three separate categories: strength, cardio, and balance. Within each category I've started off with a familiar, basic move and added three variations to it. That way you can choose from among four different versions of the same exercise, or perhaps even come up with more variations.

What's great about functional exercises is that although some focus on balance and others on strength, they all complement each other well. Some of the exercises target everything—strength, cardio, and balance—which is another reason why functional training feels complete; it always involves many interconnected parts of the body, providing you with a truly well-rounded workout.

By performing the exercises on stairs instead of on the ground, you'll encounter a different set of challenges and will work other angles. Take a look at the Plank on page 24—it becomes truly grueling when you reverse your orientation on the stairs (p. 27)!

With this type of training, there are hundreds of good exercises for you to try out.

Personally, I'm a big fan of exercises that work my entire body in several ways simultaneously, while also testing my coordination and mobility; for example, raising my shoulders while engaging my core. Or something to that effect, anyway. The beauty of functional training is that many exercises complement each other and challenge the whole entity, which may be what is the most important of all: putting our body through its paces in a way that forces us to work outside the box.

I suggest that you start by reading through the manual, and then choose a few single exercises to try out before you go for a complete exercise program.

Of course, you would be doing your body a kindness if you began each training session with an exercise from the "balance" category or walked briskly up and down the stairs a few times to elevate your heart rate. Get out there and have fun!

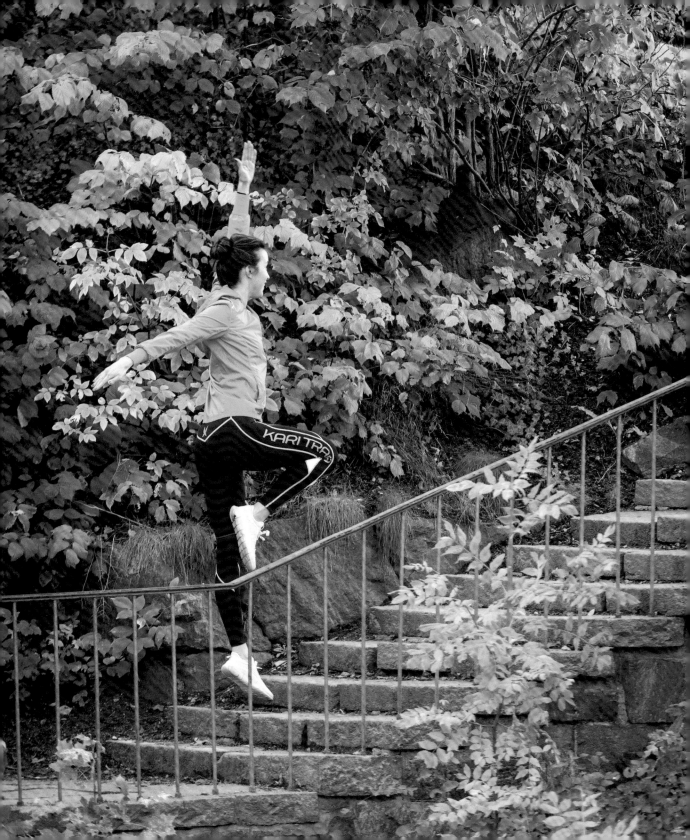

EXERCISES
STRENGTH

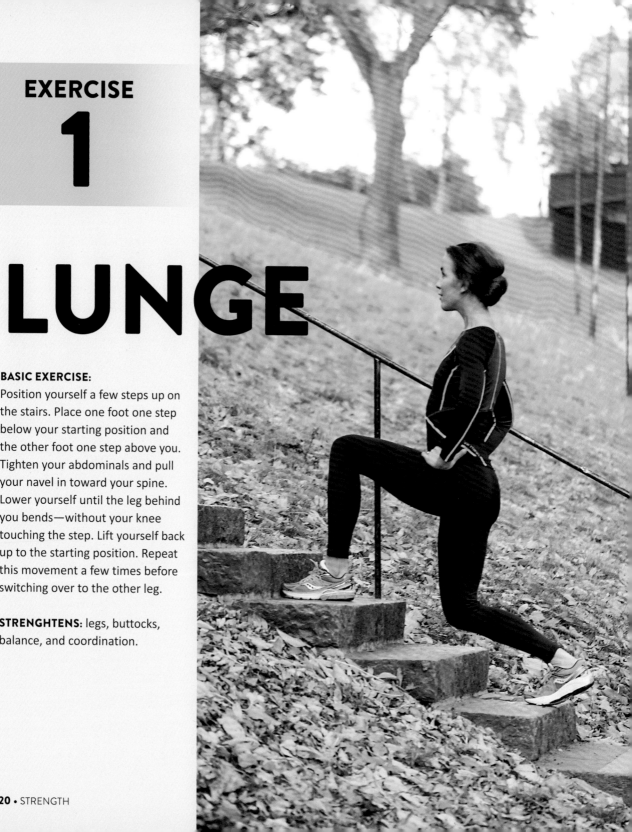

EXERCISE 1

LUNGE

BASIC EXERCISE:
Position yourself a few steps up on the stairs. Place one foot one step below your starting position and the other foot one step above you. Tighten your abdominals and pull your navel in toward your spine. Lower yourself until the leg behind you bends—without your knee touching the step. Lift yourself back up to the starting position. Repeat this movement a few times before switching over to the other leg.

STRENGHTENS: legs, buttocks, balance, and coordination.

WITH STEP-UP

Position yourself with both feet on the first step. Tighten your abdominals and pull in your navel. Take a step forward, placing your foot a few steps up, and lower your body into a lunge. Push out of the lunge and bring your legs together on the higher step, and then immediately return your leg back to the starting position on the lower step—without losing your balance and preferably without resting your foot on the step in between. Use a pendulum motion to perform the lunge—one long, smooth step up and one long, smooth step backward. Switch legs.

STRENGTHENS: thighs, buttocks, balance, and coordination.

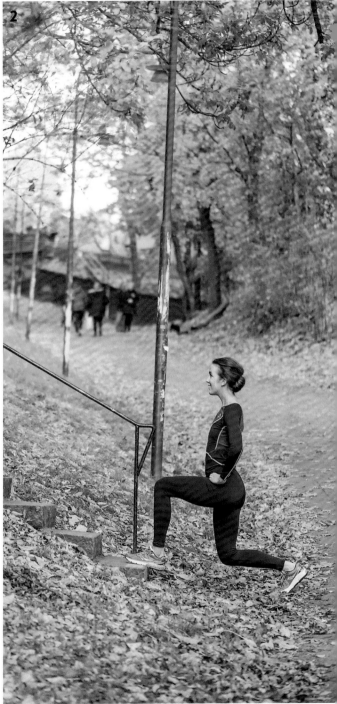

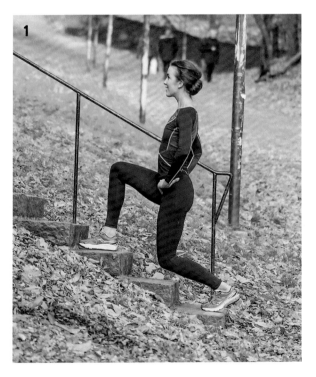

WITH UPWARD JUMP

Start from the basic position. Take a step up (like in the step-up version) but this time, push off from the foot on the higher step into an upward jump. Bring your back foot to the ground as you land and keep your front foot on the same high step. Return to the basic position and repeat. Make sure that you extend your body fully and bring your knee up toward your abdomen as you jump. Repeat several times before switching to the other leg.

STRENGTHENS: cardio, thighs, buttocks, balance, and coordination.

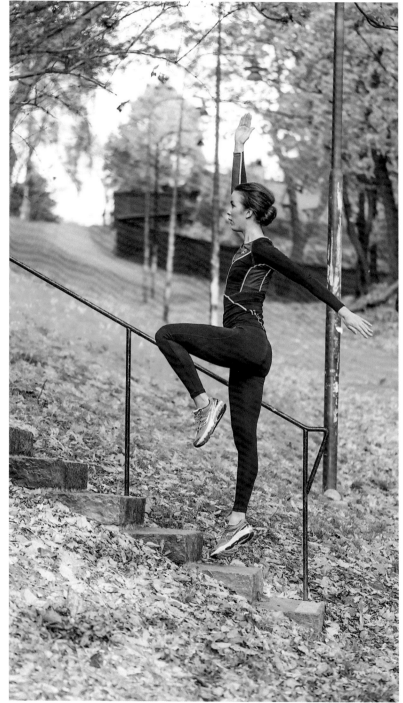

WITH LATERAL STEP

Begin with both feet on the first step, facing sideways across the steps, and crouch down into a downhill skiing position, keeping the weight in your heels, your back straight, and abdominals contracted. Push off and take a big step sideways (a few steps up), before returning to your starting position to repeat the movement. You can choose between stepping up and down or moving continually up the stairs as you step. It's important to keep your abdominals contracted and your back as straight as possible. Repeat a few times before turning and switching sides.

STRENGTHENS: thighs, buttocks, balance, and coordination.

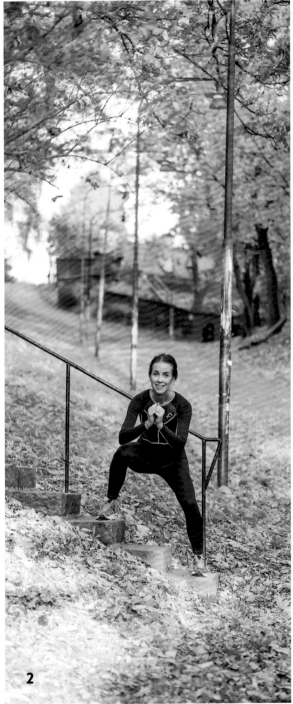

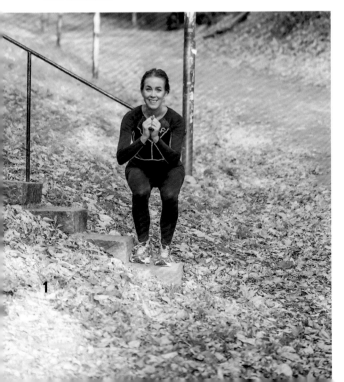

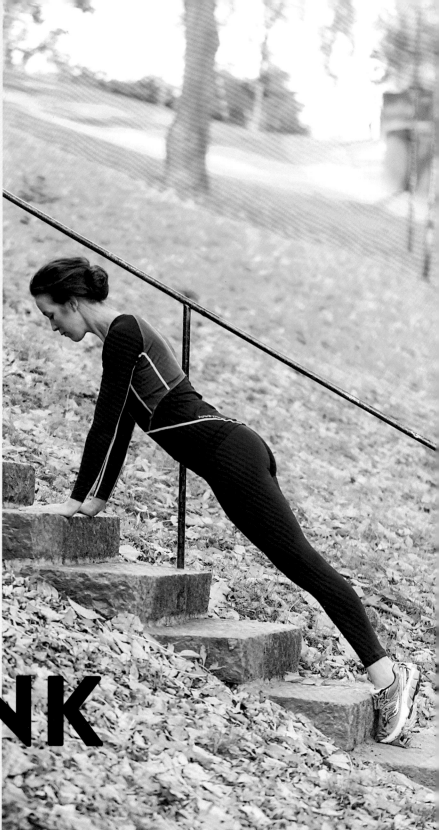

EXERCISE

2

BASIC EXERCISE:
Get into a plank position, with your arms straight and both your hands and feet on the stairs. Tighten your entire body and squeeze your glutes to pull your tailbone in between your legs, until you feel a deep, almost burning sensation within your abdominal muscles. Try to move your center of gravity back and forth a little until you locate that burning feeling. Have your neck remain as neutral as possible while your body is tense. Keep your abdominals engaged for as long as you can.

STRENGTHENS: core, shoulders, coordination, and back.

PLANK

WITH KNEE TO ELBOW

Get yourself into a basic plank position and find that burning sensation in your abdominals. When you feel the contraction in your core, slowly and carefully lift one foot off the ground, pulling your knee toward your hands. Once there, hold the position for a few seconds and then slowly return the leg to its starting position. The more slowly you perform this movement, the more challenging it will be. Alternate between each leg.

STRENGTHENS: core, shoulders, coordination, and back.

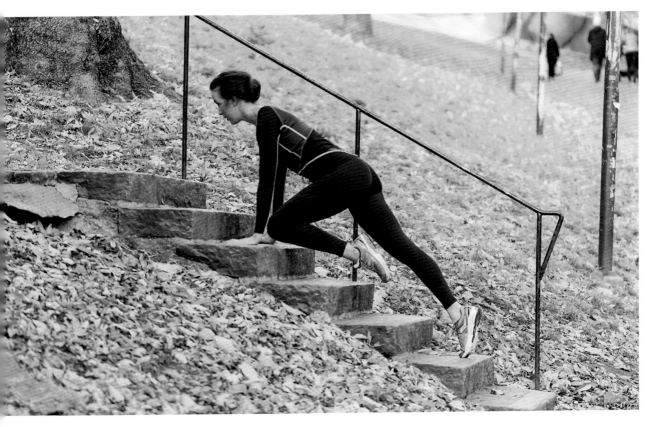

WITH A TWIST

Starting from the basic plank position, slowly pull your knee toward your chest. Carefully rotate your body sideways while staying in the plank position and maintaining that burning feeling in your abdominals. Twist your body as far as you can without compromising your form or disengaging your abdominals. Slowly return to the starting position, making sure that your hips stay straight throughout the entire exercise. Repeat on the other side.

STRENGTHENS: core, shoulders, coordination, back, and balance.

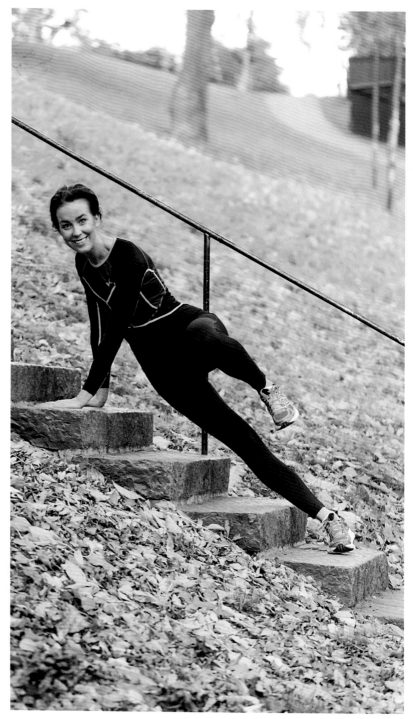

REVERSE PLANK

Start in a basic plank position but modify the exercise by reversing your body and facing "the wrong way"—toward the bottom of the stairs—with your feet on the upper step. Here you'll need to tighten your entire body and be ready, because this plank will be *significantly* harder to hold. Place most of your weight in your feet to find your stabilizing point.

STRENGTHENS: core, shoulders, wrists, cardio, and back.

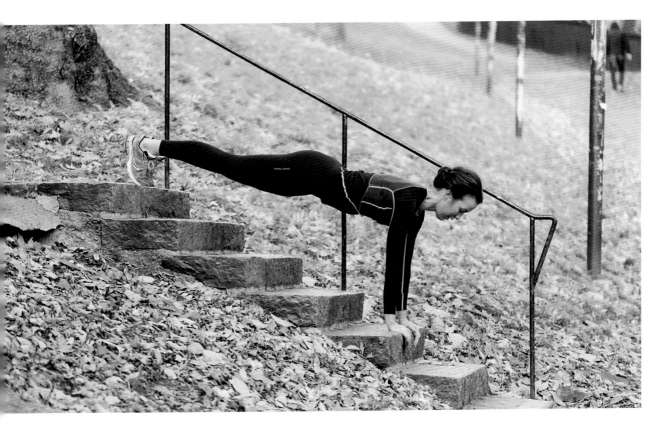

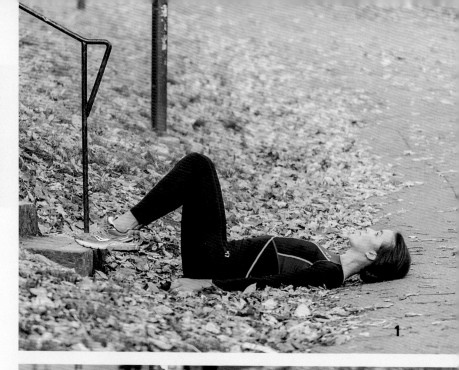

1

HIP LIFT

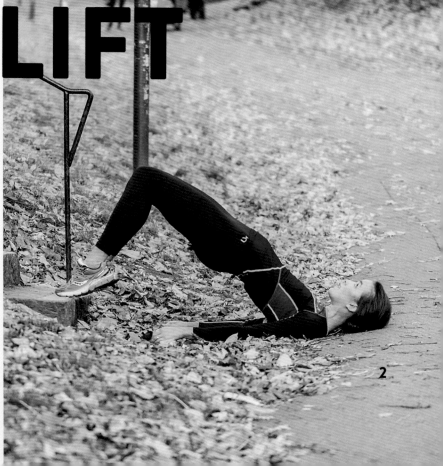

2

BASIC EXERCISE:
Lie on your back at the bottom of the stairs with your heels up on a step, your arms at your sides, and your legs bent. Raise your hips as high as you can, squeezing your buttocks hard and pushing yourself up onto your toes. Hold the position for a few seconds before slowly returning to the starting position—it's very important to control this downward motion to feel the right amount of resistance.

STRENGTHENS: back of thighs (hamstrings), buttocks, ankles, and calves.

WITH TOE RAISES

Place your feet on the first step, push your hips up as high as you can and onto your toes, as in the basic exercise. Keep your hips lifted but let your heels drop into a dip. Keep your legs tight on the way down, and then press upward again. Perform the movement in a steady rhythm.

STRENGTHENS: thighs, calves, buttocks, and coordination.

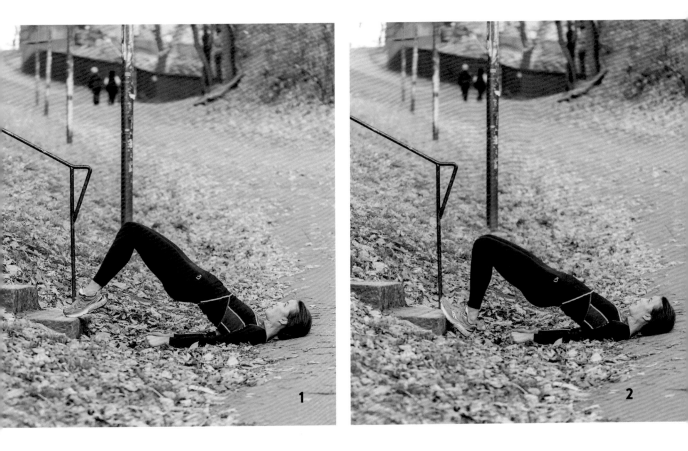

WITH LEG LIFT

Start as you would in the basic exercise but raise one leg and keep it pointed straight up throughout the entire exercise. Keep your hips level at all times. Repeat before changing leg.

STRENGTHENS: thighs, calves, ankles, buttocks, balance, and coordination.

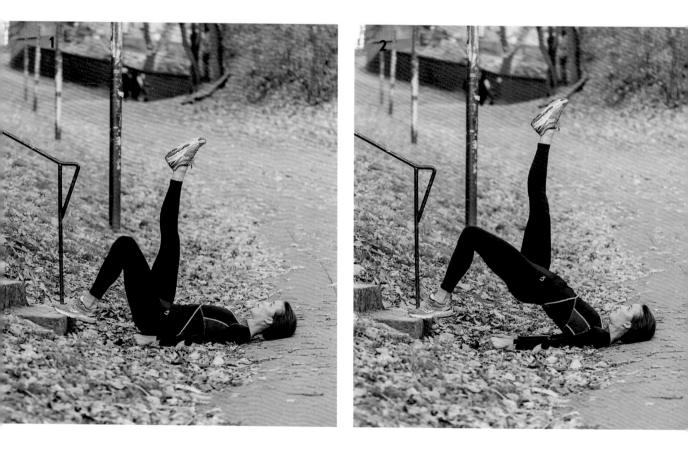

STATIC HIP BRIDGE

Start as in the basic exercise position. Push your buttocks upward and maintain this position for as long as you can. Squeeze your buttocks hard, to the point when it feels nearly impossible to hold. Remember to squeeze just that little bit harder to make it even more challenging!

STRENGTHENS: legs, buttocks, balance, coordination, core, and ankles.

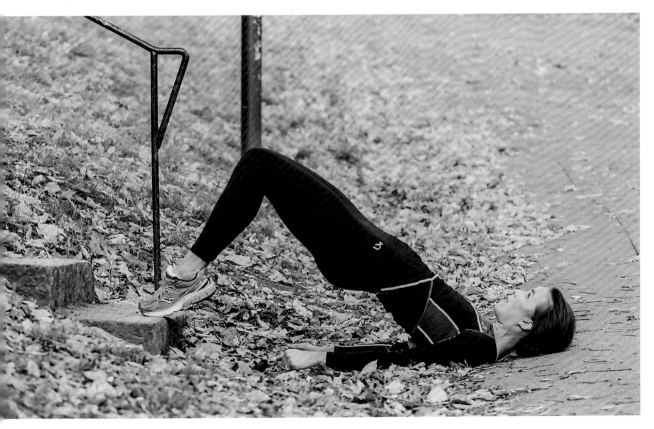

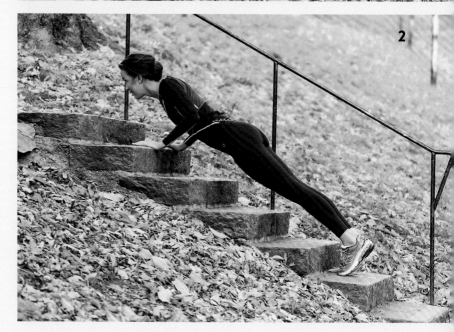

BEAR CRAWL

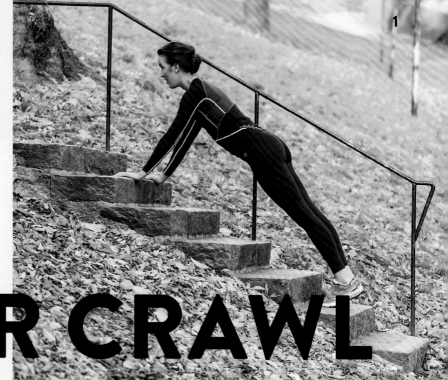

BASIC EXERCISE:
Get into the plank position, as seen on page 24. Tighten your entire body and pull your tailbone between your legs, so you get that deep, burning sensation in your abdominals. When you're in position, bend your arms a little and maintain the position.

STRENGTHENS: core, arms, legs, and buttocks.

WITH LEG LIFT

Start as in the basic exercise position, but do not bend your arms. Tighten your abdomen and bend one leg up until your toes touch the same step your hands are on. Quickly return your leg to its original position and repeat with the other leg.

STRENGTHENS: core, buttocks, arms, balance, and coordination.

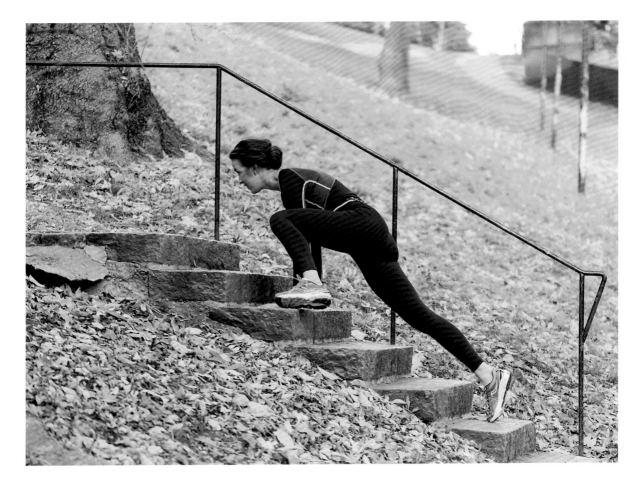

WITH FROG JUMP

Start in the basic plank position. Bend your knees, take aim, and hop up a few steps, keeping your hands on the same step. Quickly move your hands up a few steps, jump up a few more steps, and repeat until you've reached the top of the stairs. It's important to keep your abdominals contracted throughout the whole exercise.

STRENGTHENS: legs, buttocks, balance, coordination, and cardio.

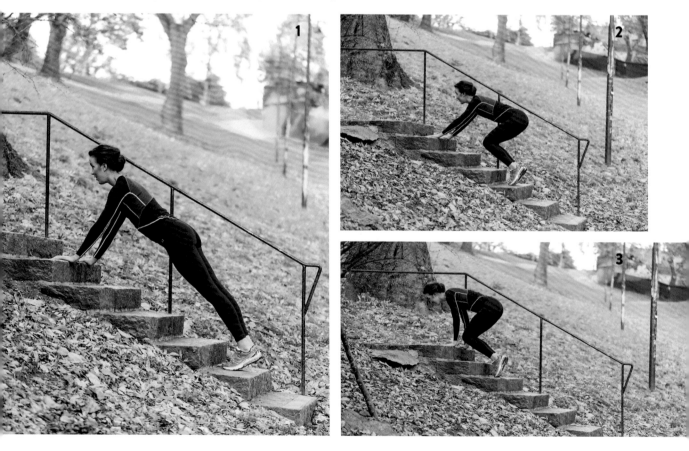

WITH JUMP

Get into the basic plank position but move your feet a few steps closer to your hands—keep your hands on the same step and your feet together throughout the entire exercise. With a hop, bring your feet a few steps up closer to your hands, and then kick your feet back to the lower starting step. It's important to keep your abdominals contracted throughout the jumps.

STRENGTHENS: arms, shoulders, balance, coordination, and core.

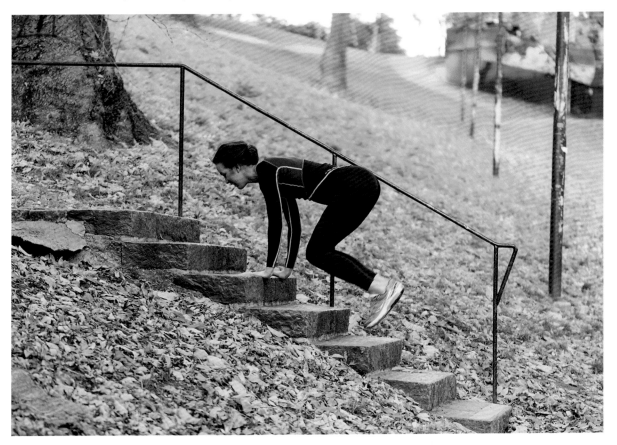

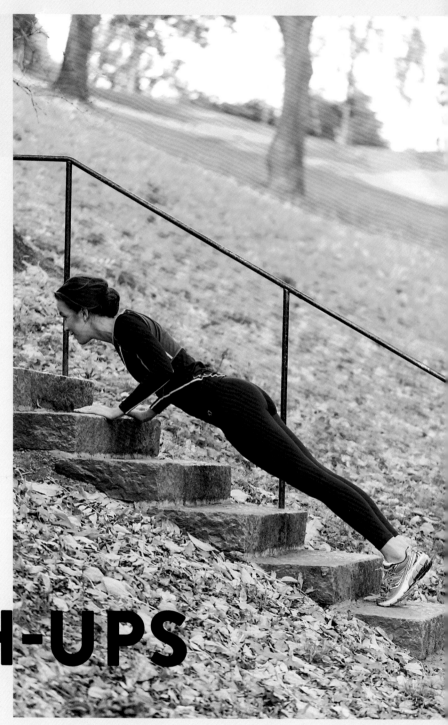

BASIC EXERCISE:
On the stairs, start in a classic push-up position with your hands shoulder-width apart. Tighten your entire body and keep your abdominals tense as in the plank exercise (see p. 24). Lower yourself slowly toward the steps by bending your arms, stopping right before touching the steps. Push back up into the starting position.

STRENGTHENS: arms, shoulders, core, and coordination.

PUSH-UPS

WITH TRICEPS FLEX

Start out in the basic position but keep your arms close to your side. Get up on your toes and bend your arms slowly. Stop when you're halfway down and hold this position for as long as you're able. Push back into starting position and repeat the exercise.

STRENGTHENS: triceps, shoulders, core, and coordination.

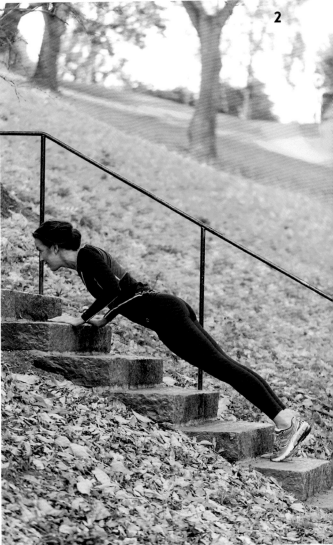

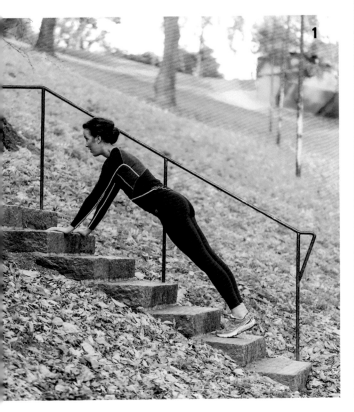

WITH ARM PUSH

Starting from the basic position, place your hands and feet so that only a few steps separate them. Contract your abdominals and push away from the steps, keeping your feet on the lower step and landing with your hands a few steps higher. Rock back and forth in short moves before pushing off from the higher step and returning your hands to the starting position. Repeat the exercise until your arms and shoulders burn.

STRENGTHENS: arms, shoulders, core, and coordination.

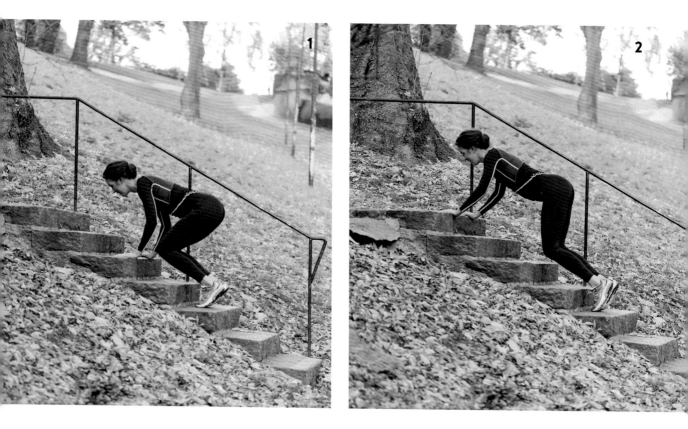

WITH WALKING PUSH-UPS

Start from the basic push-up position. Move your left arm down one step and do one push-up, then move your left arm up one step and do one push-up. Repeat the exercise with the right arm. Repeat, alternating your arms.

STRENGTHENS: arms, shoulders, core, and coordination.

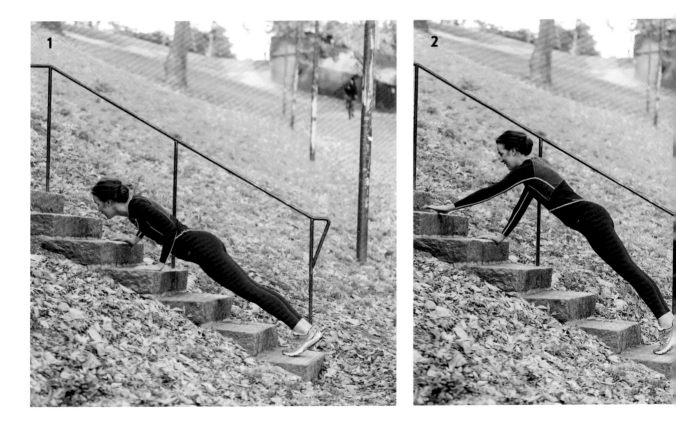

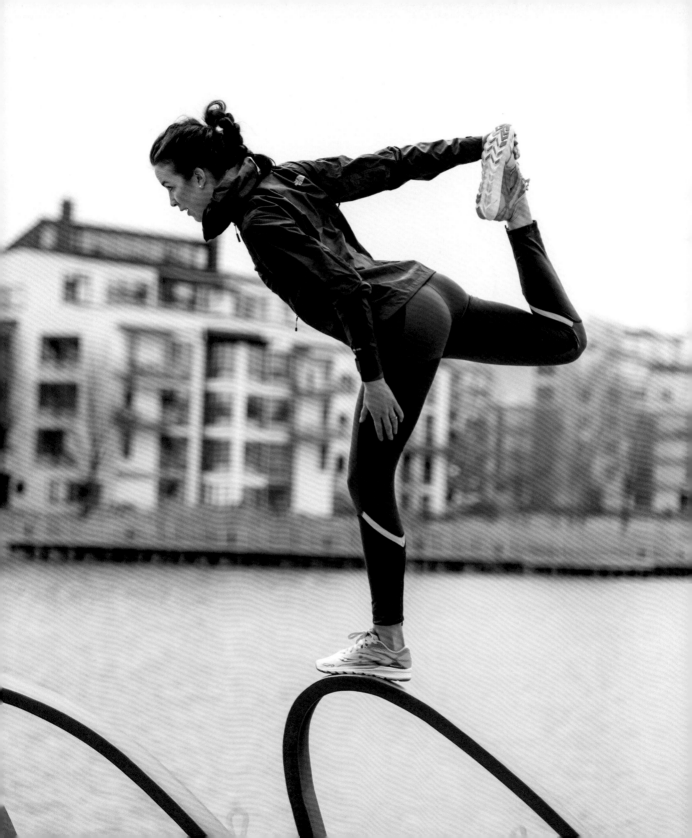

EXERCISES
BALANCE

EXERCISE
1

PENDULUM

BASIC EXERCISE:
Stand with your feet hip-width apart on a step, facing up the stairs. Start by stretching your arms over your head and slowly bend forward at the waist, keeping your hips level and back straight. Slowly lift one leg up behind you. Stop when your body makes a straight line; it will feel as if someone is pulling your hands forward and your foot backward. Slowly return to the starting position and repeat the exercise with the other leg.

STRENGTHENS: balance, coordination, back, core, and legs.

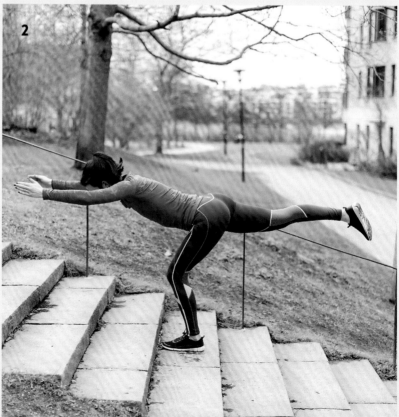

1

2

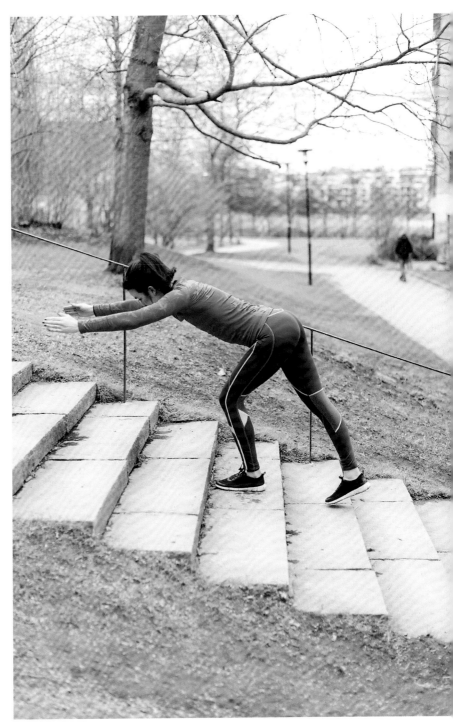

WITH TOE TAP

Start in the basic position and proceed with the exercise as seen in version 1:1. Stop when you find the balance in the pendulum with your arms and leg stretched out. Now try to tap your toes on the step below by carefully lowering your leg—without twisting your hips, bending your leg, or losing your balance. Then slowly return your leg to its outstretched position. Repeat several times before changing over to the other leg.

STRENGTHENS: thighs, buttocks, core, balance, and coordination.

WITH A YOGA TWIST

Start with the basic exercise. Stop when you've found the balance in the pendulum with your arms and leg stretched out. Try to move your arm backward and grab your foot with your hand, while carefully bending your extended leg (it's very important to use the hand that's on the same side as your foot). Stretch, and try to remain balanced and in the correct position throughout the exercise. Repeat with the other leg.

STRENGTHENS: thighs, core, balance, coordination, and ankles.

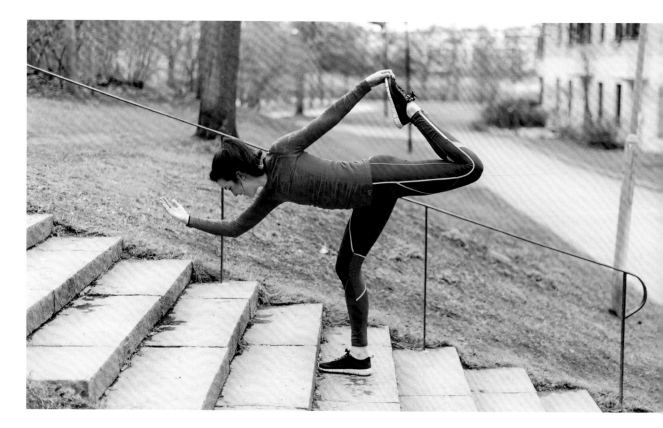

WITH HAND DIP

Start with the basic exercise and stop when you find the balance in the pendulum—with arms forward and one leg stretched out behind you. Move your arms carefully downward and try to touch the step ahead of you with your fingers (without compromising your alignment or balance), stop, and slowly return to an upright position. Change leg and repeat.

STRENGTHENS: thighs, buttocks, core, balance, coordination, and ankles.

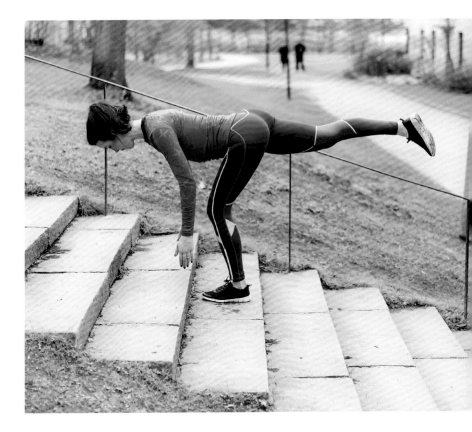

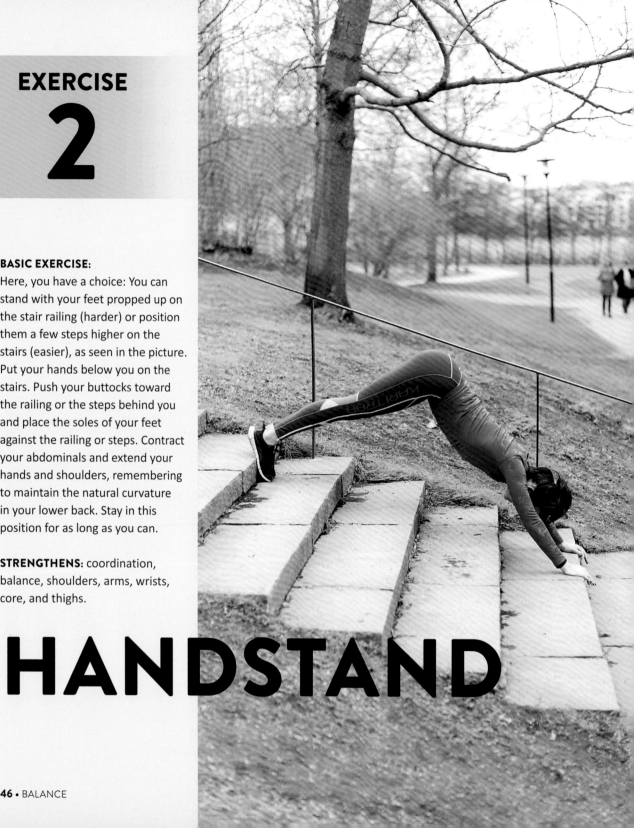

EXERCISE
2

BASIC EXERCISE:
Here, you have a choice: You can stand with your feet propped up on the stair railing (harder) or position them a few steps higher on the stairs (easier), as seen in the picture. Put your hands below you on the stairs. Push your buttocks toward the railing or the steps behind you and place the soles of your feet against the railing or steps. Contract your abdominals and extend your hands and shoulders, remembering to maintain the natural curvature in your lower back. Stay in this position for as long as you can.

STRENGTHENS: coordination, balance, shoulders, arms, wrists, core, and thighs.

HANDSTAND

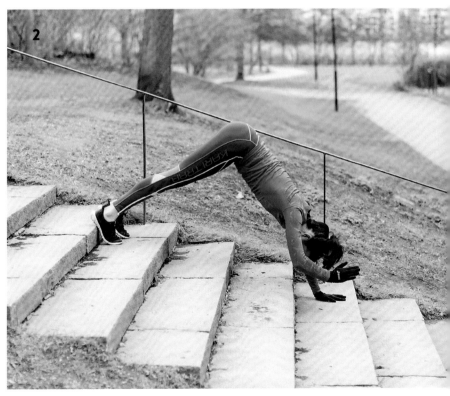

WITH HAND LIFT

Start in the basic position. When steady, carefully lift one hand a few inches off the ground and hold it there. Pay attention to your position throughout the exercise. Alternate hands.

STRENGTHENS: coordination, balance, shoulders, arms, wrists, core, and thighs.

WITH LEG LIFT

Start in the basic position—choose whether you want to do the handstand against the railing or on the stairs. Once you're steady, carefully lift one leg into the air and stretch it out above you. Hold the position for a bit by actively engaging your arms and pushing with your hands. Hold it there before switching legs.

STRENGTHENS: coordination, balance, shoulders, arms, wrists, core, and thighs.

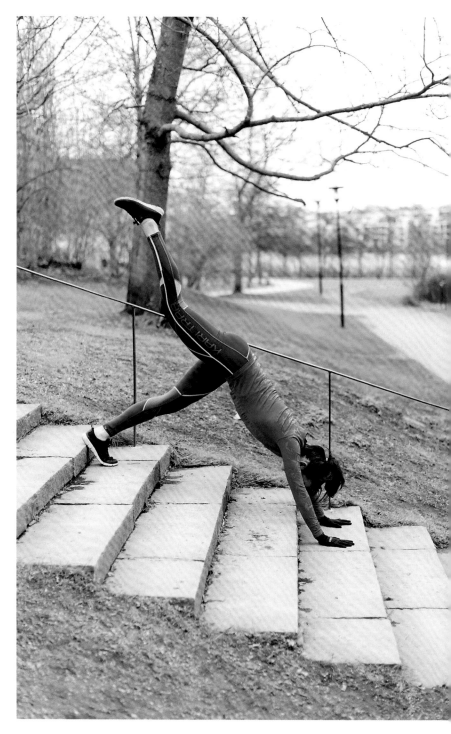

AT AN ANGLE

Start from the basic position—choose whether you want to use the railing or the steps for this exercise, which is now going to be at a sharper angle than in the basic position. Move in so that your hands are closer to your feet. Set your feet up on the railing or the step, push your body upward, and try extending your buttocks above your head. The goal is to keep your hips at a 90-degree angle. Stay in this pose for as long as you're able.

STRENGTHENS: coordination, balance, shoulders, arms, wrists, core, and thighs.

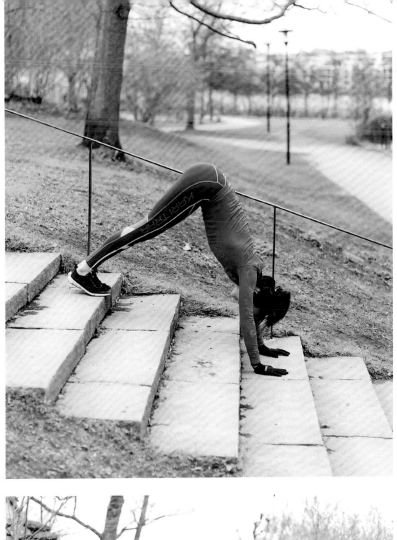

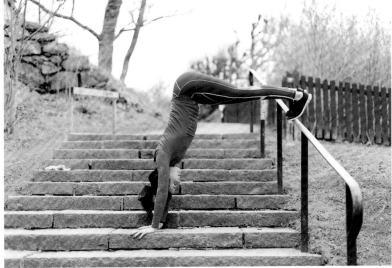

BALANCE 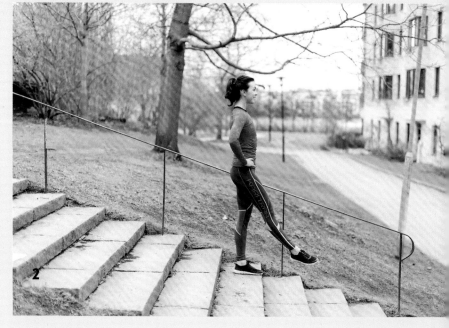 WITH LEG LIFT

BASIC EXERCISE:

Stand on the step with your left hand on the railing and look straight ahead. Contract your abdominals and straighten your posture so it's upright and strong. Pull your abdominals in to neutralize the curvature of your lower back. As you exhale, lift your right leg (maybe only by an inch or two to begin with) in front of you, taking care not to compromise your posture. Hold your leg up for a few seconds before slowly lowering it back down again. Repeat this movement a few times before switching to the other leg.

STRENGTHENS: legs, core, coordination, balance, and ankles.

WITH LATERAL RAISE

This is like the basic position, except you will now lift your leg out to the side. Try to lift it without compromising your posture or changing your position. Hold your leg up for a few seconds before slowly lowering it down. Repeat the movement a few times before you switch over to the other leg.

STRENGTHENS: core, legs, buttocks, coordination, balance, and ankles.

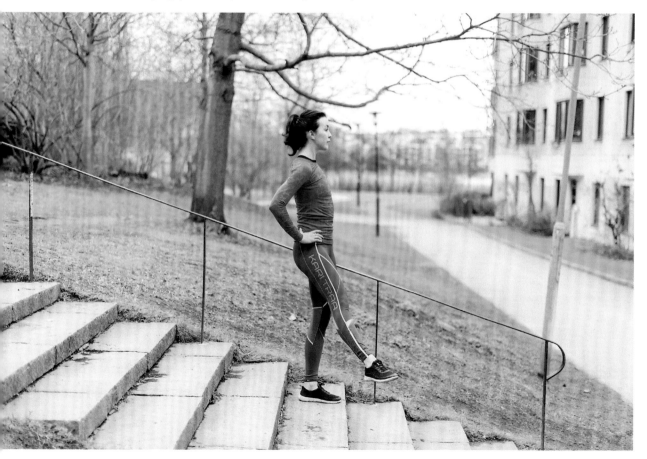

WITH TOE LIFT

Start as in the basic exercise, but once you've extended your leg, exhale further and push yourself onto your toes. Strive to keep your balance and to not modify your position. Keep your leg in the air for a few seconds before slowly lowering it to the starting point. Repeat the movement a few times before switching over to the other leg.

STRENGTHENS: core, coordination, balance, thighs, calves, and ankles.

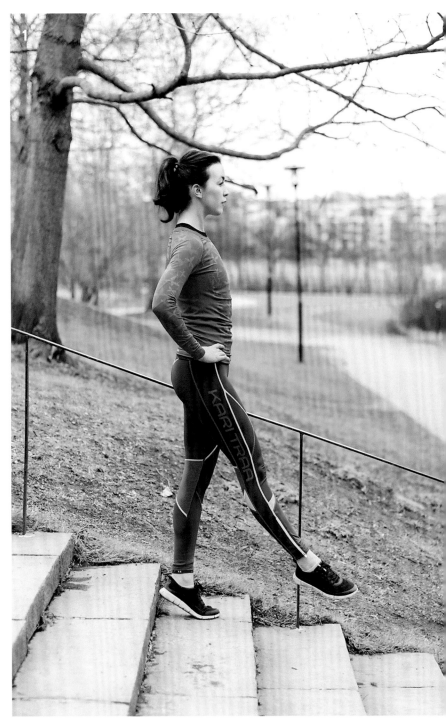

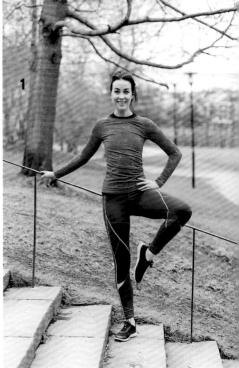

WITH SIDEWAYS PENDULUM

Start with your back against the railing. Hold on to the railing with one hand if you need to. Lift one leg and slowly bend sideways in the opposite direction, as far as you can go without losing your balance or compromising your form. Slowly return to the starting point and repeat with the other leg.

STRENGTHENS: core, thighs, coordination, balance, and ankles.

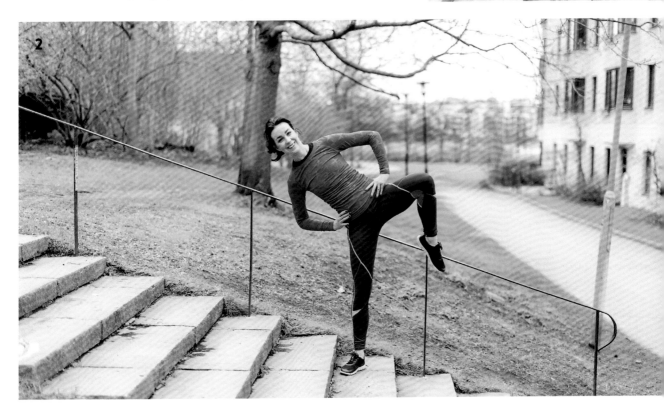

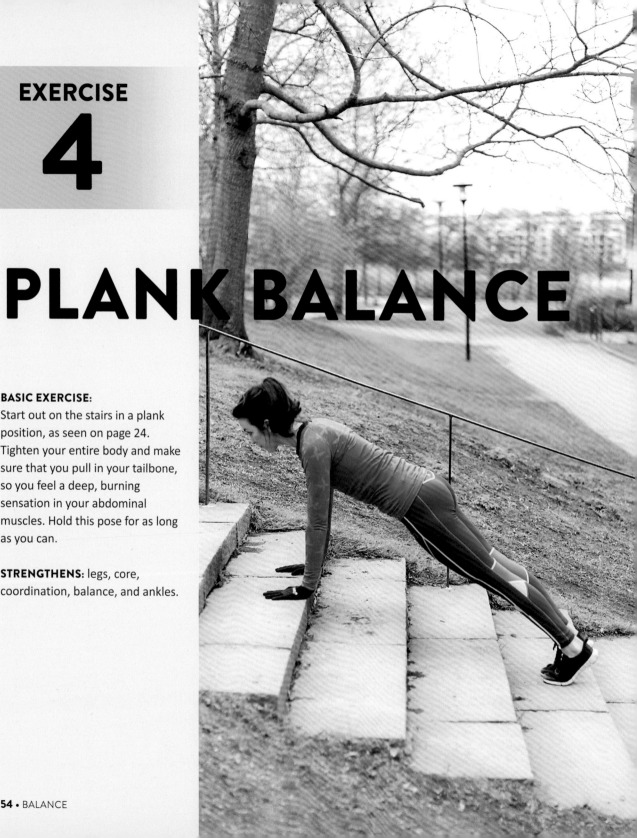

PLANK BALANCE

BASIC EXERCISE:
Start out on the stairs in a plank position, as seen on page 24. Tighten your entire body and make sure that you pull in your tailbone, so you feel a deep, burning sensation in your abdominal muscles. Hold this pose for as long as you can.

STRENGTHENS: legs, core, coordination, balance, and ankles.

WITH SIDE PLANK

Start in the basic position. Rotate carefully until you get into a side plank position, with only one foot and one hand on the stairs. Contract your abdominals, keep your hips straight, and stretch your other arm up over your head. Keep this position as steady and for as long as you can manage, preferably for 20 to 30 seconds, before switching sides.

STRENGTHENS: core, balance, shoulders, and coordination.

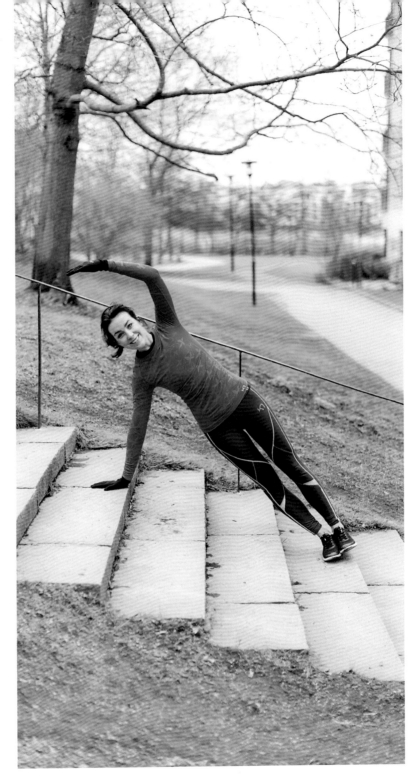

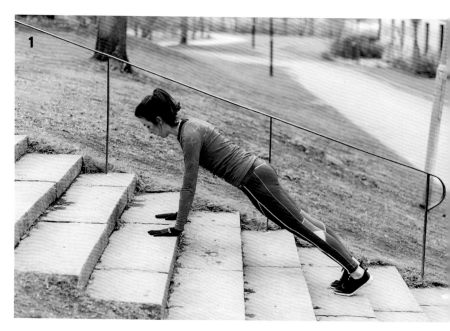

WITH ROTATION

Perform the same movement as in the last exercise, except this time, keep moving. Start in the plank position, then rotate slowly over to a side plank. Find your balance, then rotate back to the basic plank. Repeat the side plank, but on the other side.

STRENGTHENS: core, balance, shoulders, and coordination.

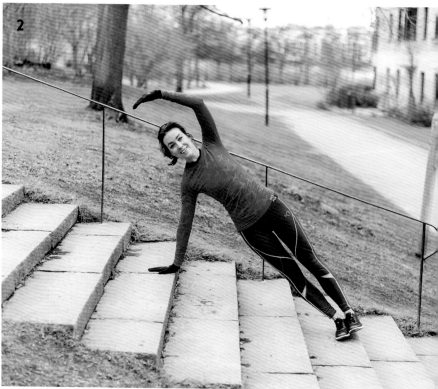

WITH BACKWARD BEND

Sit down on a step, your feet hip-width apart on a step farther down and your hands on the step just above the one you're sitting on. Push your hips up skyward and slowly let your head lean back. If you want to, and can, try slowly lifting a leg without dropping your hips or losing your balance. Stay in this pose for a bit before switching legs or returning to the starting position.

STRENGTHENS: core, balance, shoulders, coordination, and legs.

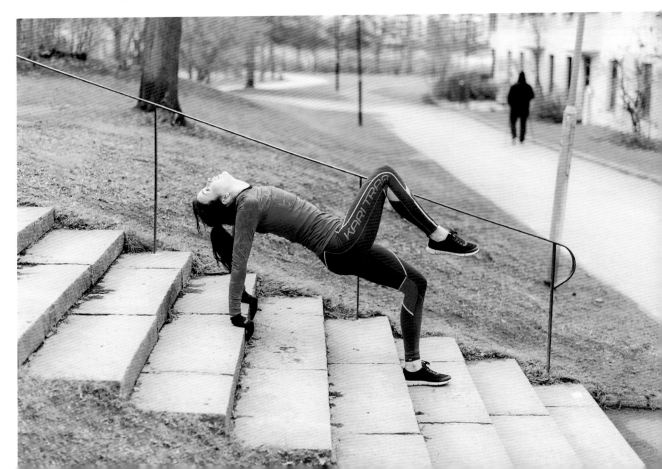

EXERCISE
5

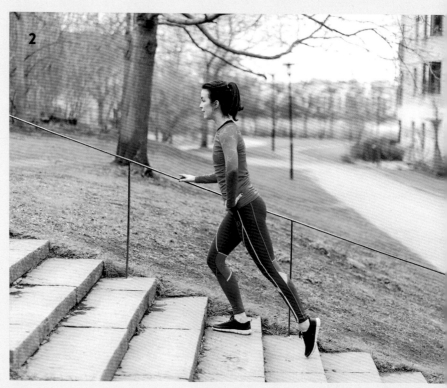

BALANCE WITH STEP

BASIC EXERCISE:
Stand at the middle point of the stairs, with your hand on the railing if needed. Tighten your abdominals and stretch your body to feel it engage. Slowly lift your leg to the step above and tap it with your toes, then slowly move your foot down to the step below and tap your toes on that step before returning to the starting position. Do this exercise slowly to focus on your balance and strength. Keep your abdominals contracted throughout the movement. Repeat it a few times before switching over to the other leg.

STRENGTHENS: thighs, core, balance, and coordination.

WITH DOWNWARD STEP

Start in the basic position but try to extend your foot 2 or 3 steps farther down. Shift your weight to your heels and bend forward slightly. Perform the exercise slowly, bending your front leg a little to reach and tapping the lower step before returning to starting position. Repeat the movement a few times before switching over to the other leg.

STRENGTHENS: thighs, buttocks, balance, and coordination.

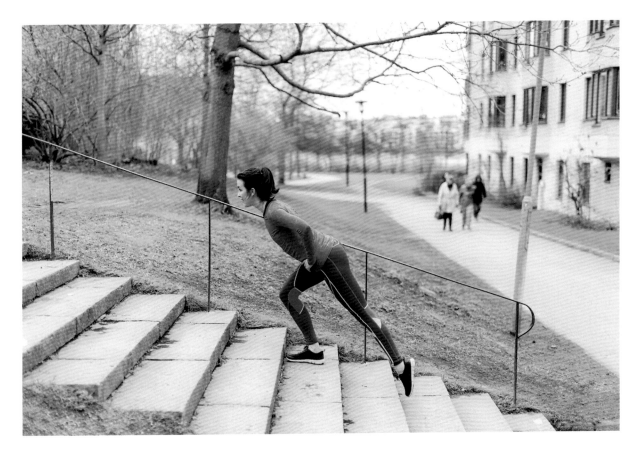

WITH STEP-UP

Stand with your back to the steps. Perform the basic exercise but lift your leg a little so you can stretch it behind you and touch a step above you with your foot. Do this exercise slowly and keep your abdominals contracted throughout. Switch legs and repeat.

STRENGTHENS: thighs, buttocks, balance, and coordination.

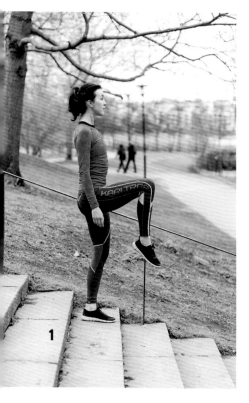

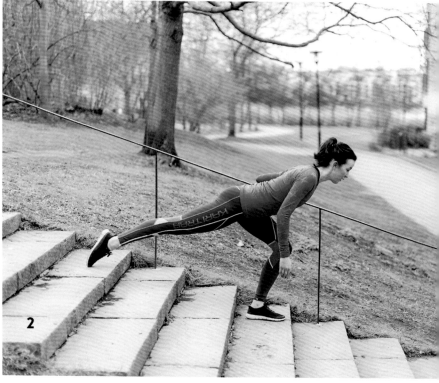

WITH LATERAL STEP

Stand sideways on the stairs with your back against the railing, and your hand on the railing if needed. Contract your abdominals, bend your right leg slightly, and step down 1 to 3 steps with your left foot. Let your foot just graze the lower step and push yourself back up again. Repeat the move a few times before switching over to the other leg.

STRENGTHENS: thighs, buttocks, balance, and coordination.

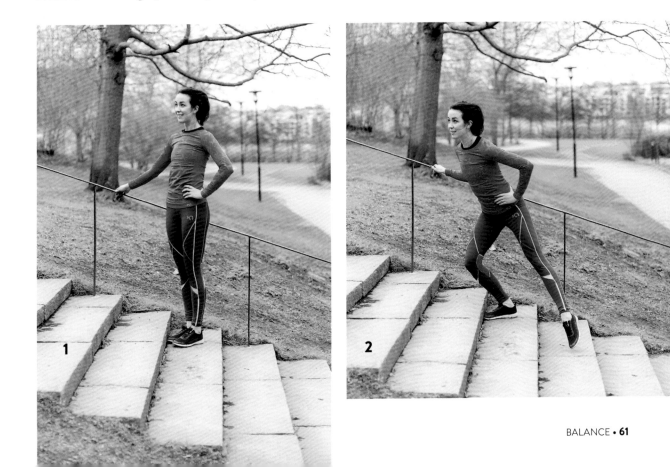

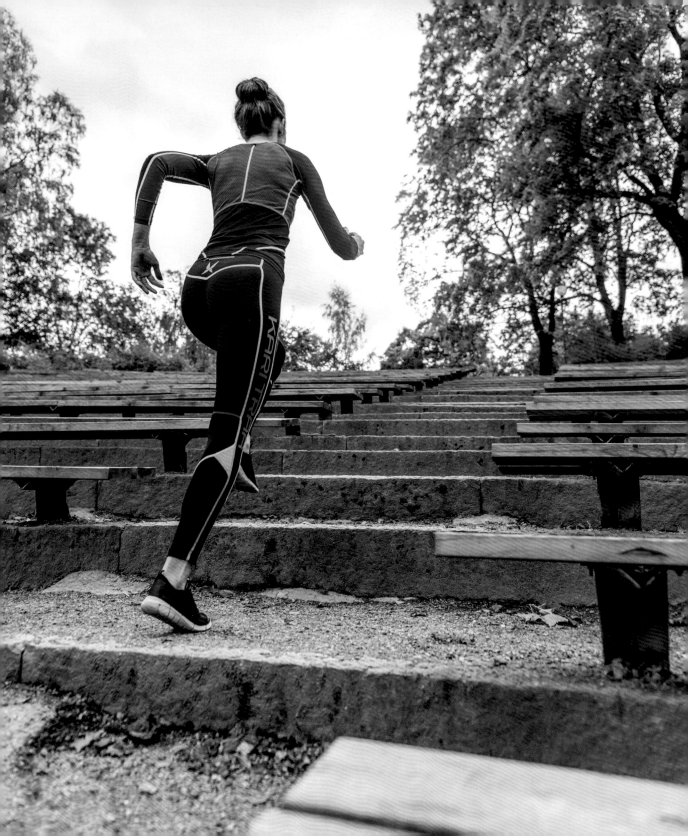

EXERCISES
CARDIO

1

BASIC EXERCISE:
Stand at the foot of the stairs, with your feet hip-width apart. Bend your legs as if you were going to do a squat, with your weight centered in your heels. Jump up onto the first step. If you feel strong, jump back down to the starting position; otherwise, just step down.

STRENGTHENS: cardio, thighs, buttocks, and coordination.

STAIR JUMPS

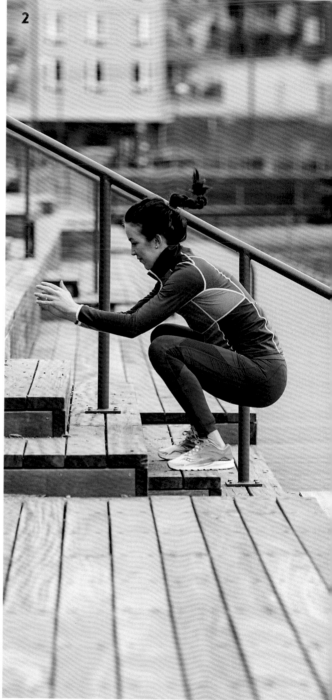

WITH VERTICAL JUMP

Start in the basic position but continue jumping up the entire flight of stairs, preferably without stopping. It's very important to keep your abdominals engaged and to make the jumps seamless.

STRENGTHENS: cardio, legs, buttocks, balance, and coordination.

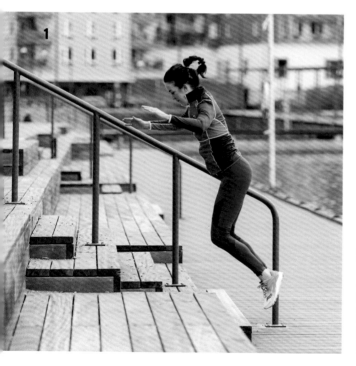

WITH LATERAL JUMP

Stand at the foot of the stairs with your hip facing the stairs. With your feet hip-width apart, bend your knees as in a squat, with your weight centered in your heels. Jump or step sideways all the way up the stairs as if you were running a lateral steeplechase. Switch sides and repeat.

STRENGTHENS: cardio, legs, buttocks, balance, and coordination

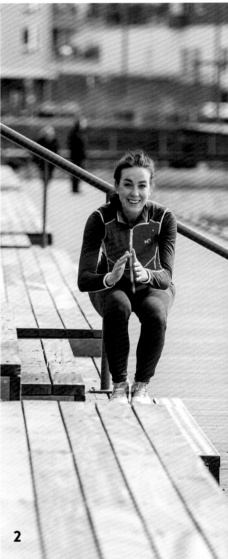

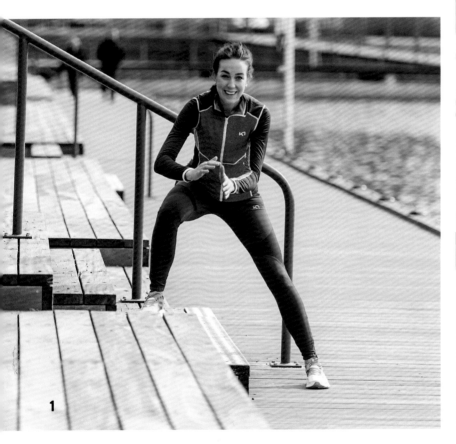

WITH LONG JUMP

Start in the basic position. Now aim to reach a few steps up and jump as many of them as you can. Quickly step down to the starting point and repeat. Vary between jumping 1, 2, 3, and maybe even 4 steps at a time, to work cardio and strength, as well as bravery.

STRENGTHENS: cardio, thighs, buttocks, balance, coordination.

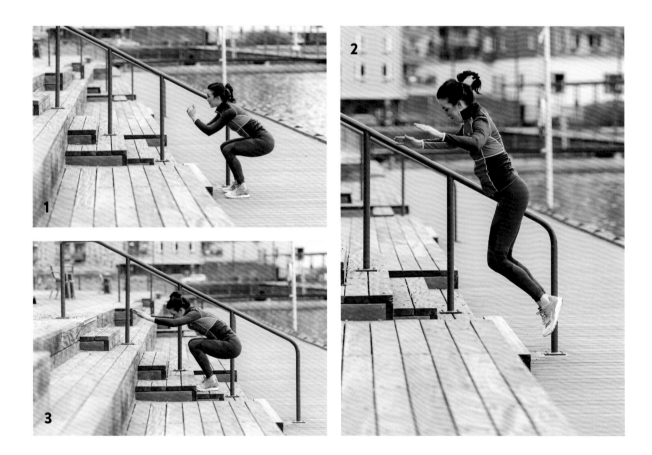

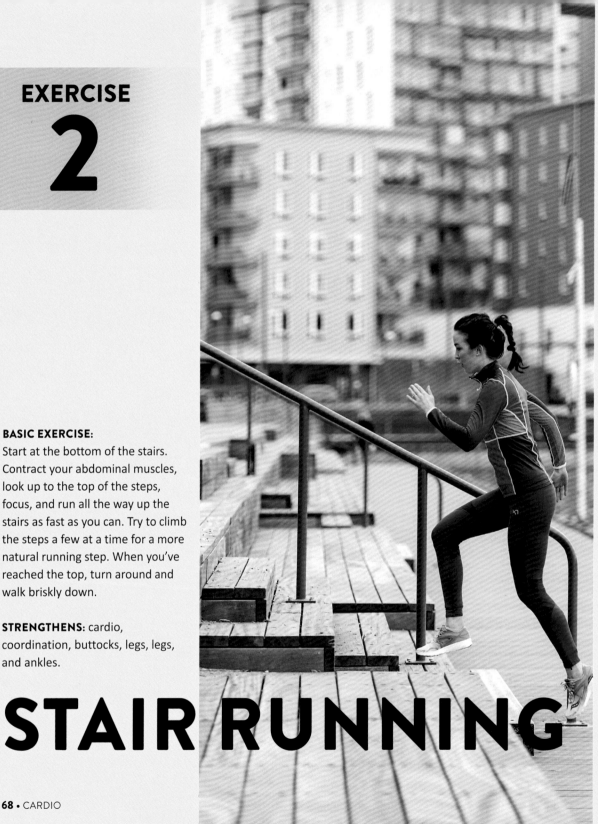

EXERCISE

2

BASIC EXERCISE:
Start at the bottom of the stairs.
Contract your abdominal muscles,
look up to the top of the steps,
focus, and run all the way up the
stairs as fast as you can. Try to climb
the steps a few at a time for a more
natural running step. When you've
reached the top, turn around and
walk briskly down.

STRENGTHENS: cardio,
coordination, buttocks, legs, legs,
and ankles.

STAIR RUNNING

WITH QUICK STEP-UPS

Do the basic exercise but concentrate on hitting every step on the way up.
Lift your knees and run as fast as you can up the stairs.

STRENGTHENS: cardio, legs, buttocks, balance, and coordination.

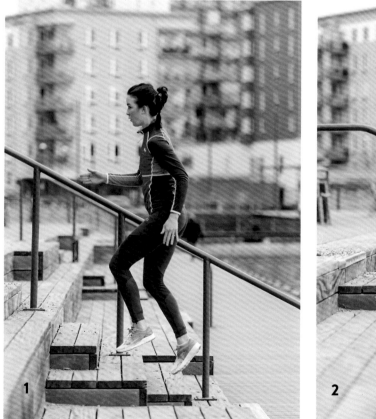

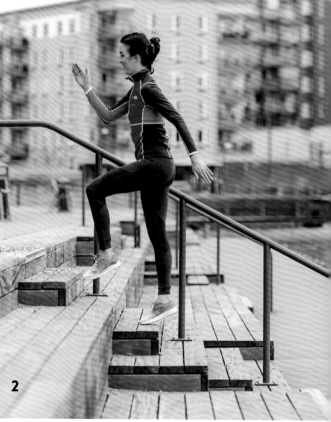

WITH HIGH KNEE STEP-UPS

Perform the basic exercise, but quickly lift your knees as high as you can while you do it.

STRENGTHENS: legs, buttocks, balance, and coordination.

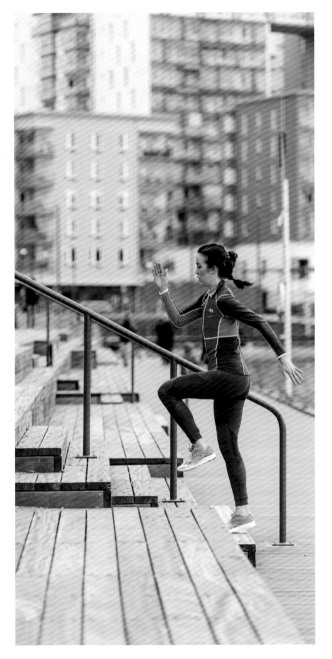

JUMP WITH DOUBLE ARM SWING

Run to the top of the stairs while lifting your knees high and swinging your arms. Contract your abdominal muscles and be careful where you put your feet.

STRENGTHENS: legs, buttocks, balance, and coordination

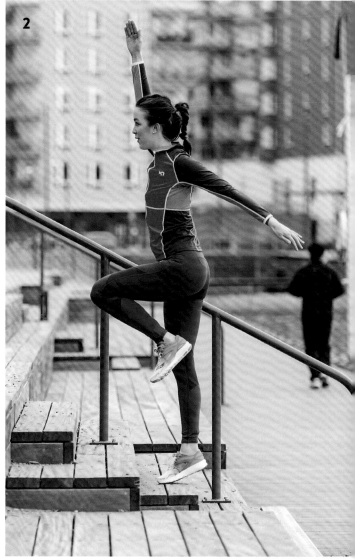

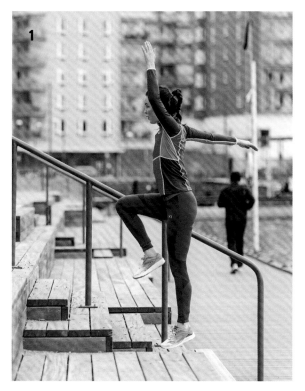

EXERCISE
3

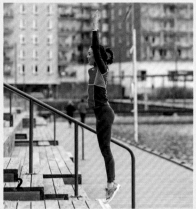

BURPEE

BASIC EXERCISE:
Start by standing on the bottom step. Squat down to a sitting position and jump up a step while lifting your arms over your head, then immediately place your hands 2 steps up. Kick your feet and legs back down a few steps to a standing plank. Jump back to the seated squat position. From there, jump straight up, bringing your arms up and over your head.

STRENGTHENS: cardio, coordination, shoulders, core, thighs, and buttocks.

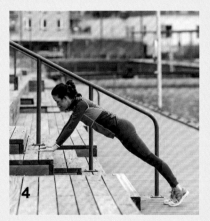

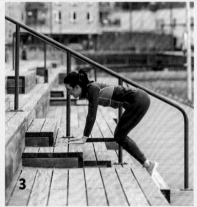

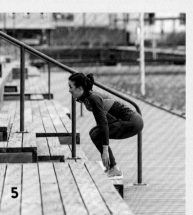

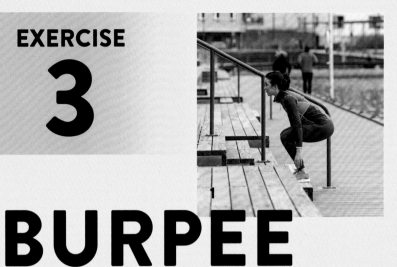

CLIMBING BURPEES

Stand on the first step of the stairs and jump up. When you land, bend forward and place your hands on the step above your feet and start climbing a few steps with your hands. Your feet stay in the same place during the hand climb. Once you reach the plank position, climb back down with your hands to the original position, then jump up again. Repeat the exercise all the way up the stairs.

STRENGTHENS: cardio, thighs, buttocks, balance, and coordination.

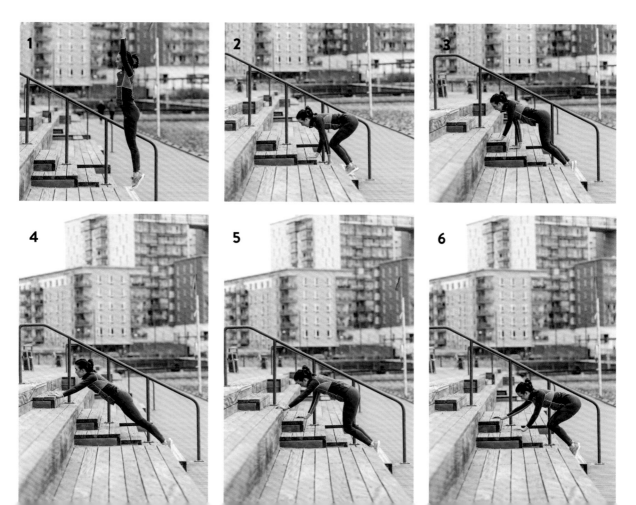

WALKING BURPEE

Perform the basic exercise, but in this version, everything is done while walking. You walk back one step at a time rather than jumping back, and instead of jumping up, you stretch your arms quickly overhead. By "walking" through the burpee it's easier to reach a pace that will raise your heart rate.

STRENGTHENS: fitness, legs, buttocks, balance, and coordination.

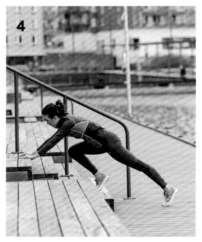

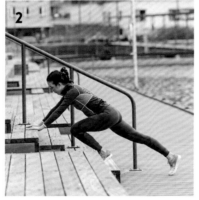

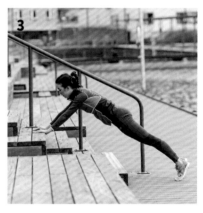

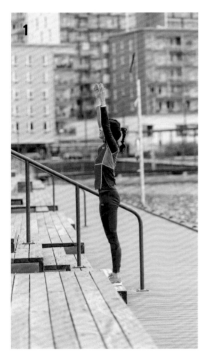

BURPEE PUSH-UPS

Perform the basic burpee, but when you get to the plank position, do a push-up before returning to the starting position.

STRENGTHENS: cardio, legs, buttocks, balance, and coordination.

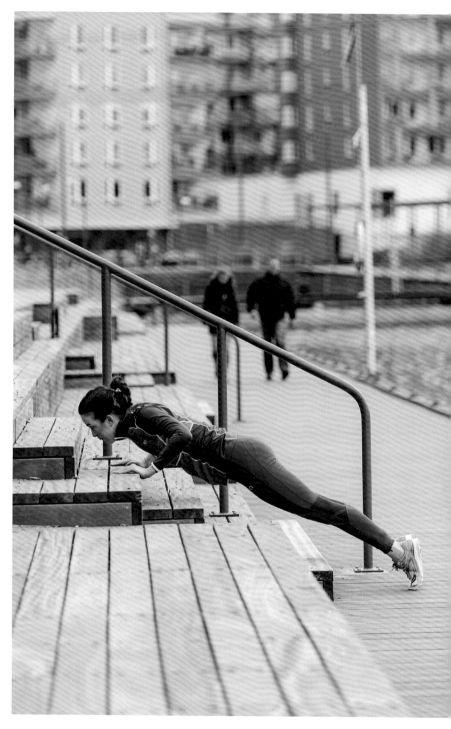

BASIC EXERCISE:
The basic position for this exercise is identical to that of the Stair Running exercise on page 68.

STRENGTHENS: cardio, coordination, legs, ankles, and core.

INTERVAL TRAINING

THE CLASSIC

Start with the basic exercise but try to increase your speed a bit as you approach the top of the stairs, then walk down quickly. Repeat 10 times. Try to find a challenging set of stairs for this one!

STRENGTHENS: cardio, legs, buttocks, balance, and coordination.

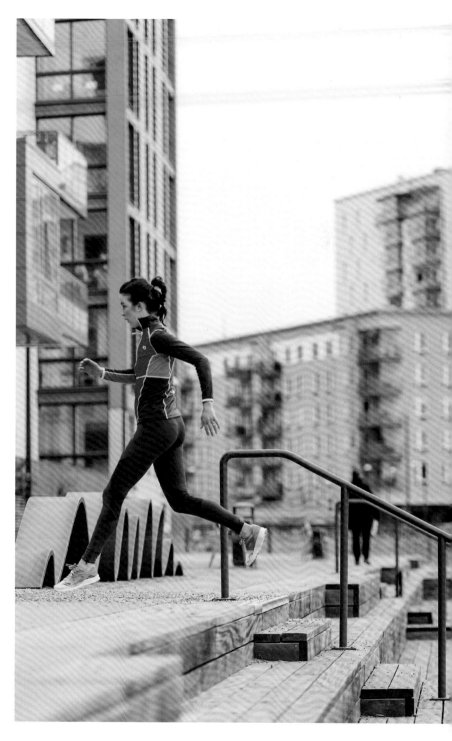

THE DUMMY

The Dummy is a classic exercise where you run up a few steps, run back down, run up a bit farther, then come back down again, and repeat until you've made it all the way to the top of the stairs. Increase your effort by doing 3 to 4 steps at a time. Avoid running down the stairs if you have sensitive knees. Instead, run up as fast as you can, and then walk down.

STRENGTHENS: cardio, legs, buttocks, balance, and coordination.

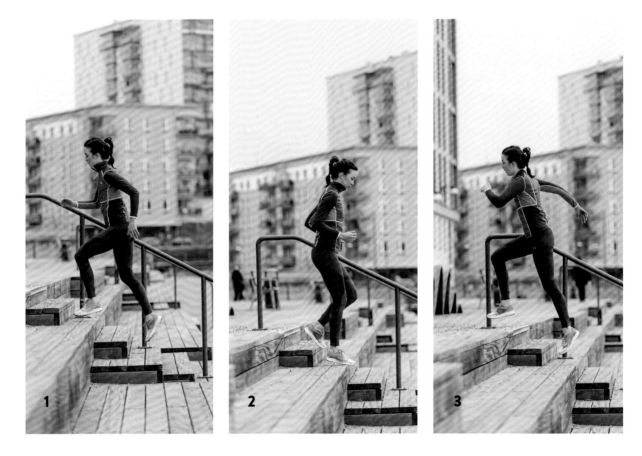

WITH BOUNCY STEPS

Start from the basic position but add some bounce to your running step to work on your stamina. Move so quickly that you can push and bounce off with your foot to the next step—like how a triple-jump athlete runs at the end of the approach. Run up fast and walk quickly down.

STRENGTHENS: cardio, legs, buttocks, balance, and coordination.

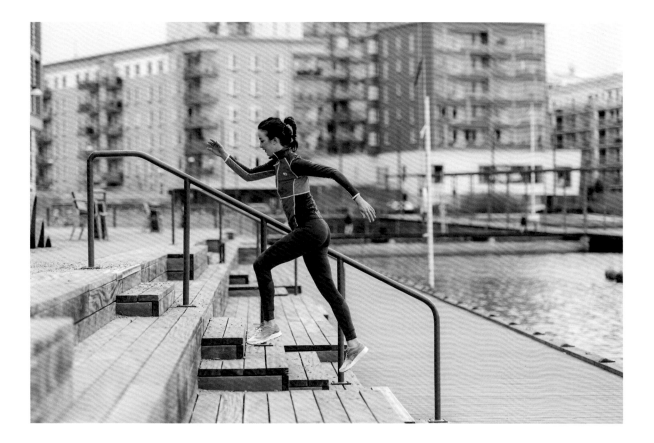

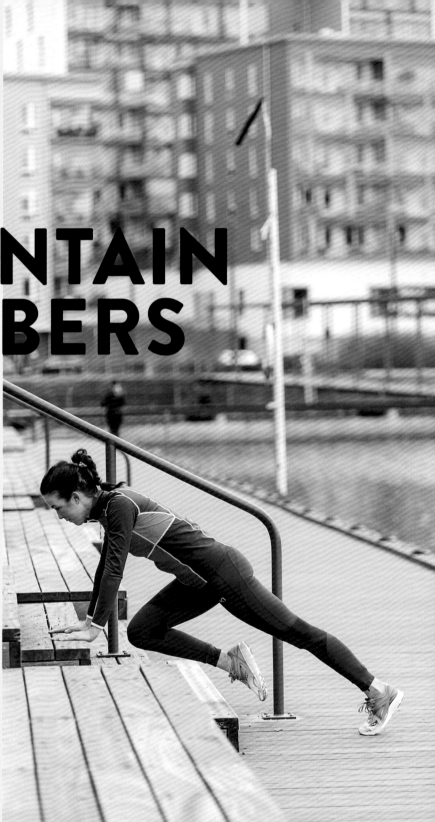

5

MOUNTAIN CLIMBERS

BASIC EXERCISE:
Put your hands on the second step of the stairs and place your body in the plank position, engaging your abdominals until you feel them burn (see p. 24). Contracting your abdominals, pull up each leg alternately toward your elbows.

STRENGTHENS: cardio, coordination, core, arms, and legs.

WITH BIKE RUN

Start out in the basic position. This time you'll "run" by rapidly pulling up your legs alternately toward the outside of your arms.

STRENGTHENS: cardio, legs, buttocks, balance, and coordination.

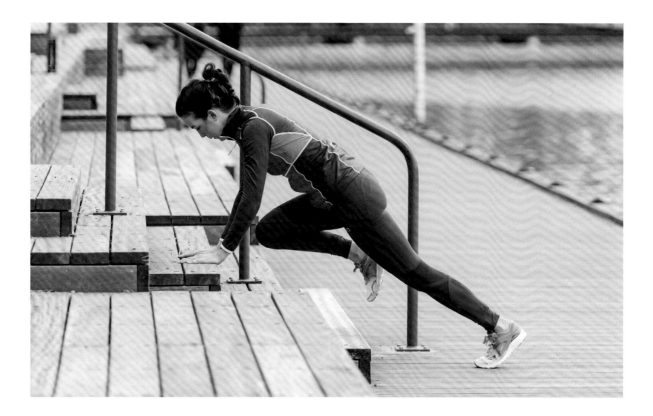

WITH RUNNING HANDS

Place yourself in the plank position with your feet on the first step and your hands a few steps up. Instead of pulling up your knees as in the basic exercise, "run" your hands up and down the nearest steps. Keep your core engaged and your feet firmly on the first step.

STRENGTHENS: cardio, legs, buttocks, balance, and coordination.

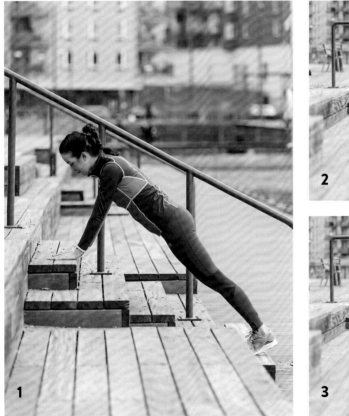

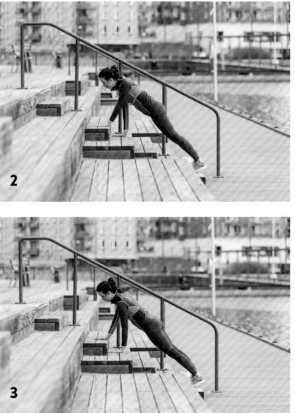

WITH PENDULUM

Start in the basic position, but instead of pulling up your knees, jump while alternating your legs' positions on the steps. If you are able, try to line your front foot up with your hands. Try to create a pace at which your legs switch back and forth at quick speed.

STRENGTHENS: cardio, legs, buttocks, balance, and coordination.

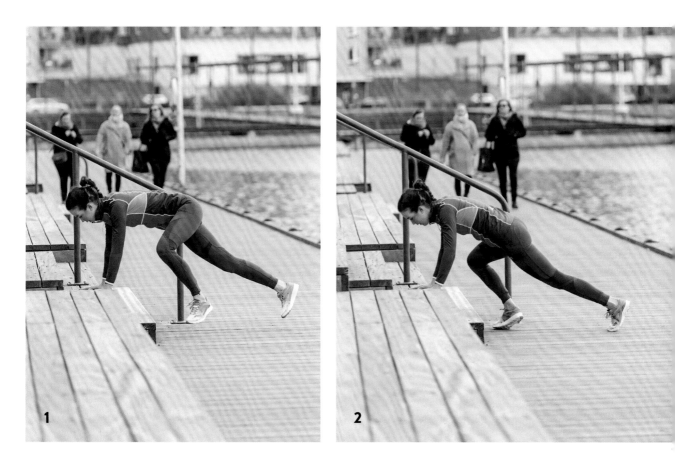

1

2

EXERCISE PROGRAMS

• Time spent on each session does not include a warm-up.

HEART RATE BOOSTER

• **TIME:** 5 minutes
• **EXERCISES:** *Mountain Climbers 1* and *Mountain Climbers 3*
• **WARM-UP:** *Stair Running*
• **HOW TO:** Before you begin, download the app "Tabata timer." Engage in your choice of warm-up activity for 1 to 2 minutes. Then do the exercises Tabata-style: 8 sets of exercises at 20 seconds per set with 10-second rests, alternating between exercises. Finish off with 1 minute of stair running, doing whichever version you like. This is an opportunity for you to go all-out in a very effective way. *Go! Go!*

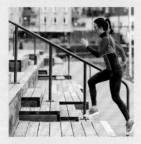

• Warm-up
Stair Running (p. 68)

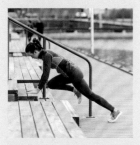

1. Mountain Climbers 1 (p. 81)

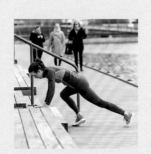

2. Mountain Climbers 3 (p. 83)

IN-MOTION WORKOUT

• **TIME:** 5 minutes
• **EXERCISES:** *Pendulum, Pendulum 2, Bear Crawl 1*
• **WARM-UP:** *Burpee*
• **HOW TO:** Warm up with Burpee 2. Do 6 to 10 reps of this exercise to get started. Then perform each exercise for 1 minute and 40 seconds. Do one exercise at a time. Concentrate on doing the exercise using proper form, and don't stress out over it. You have time to do much more than you imagine.

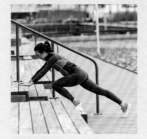

• Warm-up
Burpee 2 (p. 74)

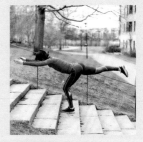

1. Pendulum (p. 42)

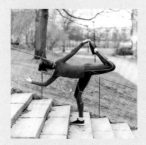

2. Pendulum 2 (p. 44)

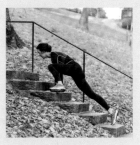

3. Bear Crawl 1 (p. 33)

QUICK FULL-BODY CHALLENGE

- **TIME:** 5 minutes
- **EXERCISES:** *Mountain Climbers 3* and *Stair Jump 3*
- **WARM-UP:** *Stair Running*
- **HOW TO:** Download the app "Tabata timer." Choose your warm-up and do it for 1 to 2 minutes. Then do the exercises Tabata-style: 8 sets of exercises at 20 seconds per set with 10 second rests, alternating between exercises. Finish off with 1 minute of stair running, whichever version you like. This routine is a perfect heart-rate booster with which to cap off your walk!

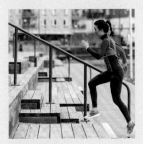

- Warm-up
Stair Running (p. 68)

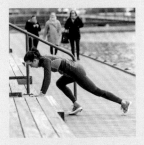

1. Mountain Climbers 3 (p. 83)

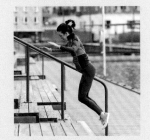

2. Stair Jump 3 (p. 67)

CORE FOCUS

- **TIME:** 5 minutes
- **EXERCISES:** *Plank* (or *Plank 2* if you want more of a challenge) and *Push-ups 3*
- **WARM-UP:** *Pendulum*
- **HOW TO:** Warm up with Pendulum. Perform 5 to 6 reps, or until you are in touch with your body and you feel ready. Set a timer for 5 minutes and use these minutes to challenge yourself. Remain in the plank position for as long as you can—to the point where it feels impossible to stay in position one more second—and then see if you can't count down from three and make the plank last just a little bit longer. Take a short break for 5 to 10 seconds. Then do the same with the push-ups: engage your abdominals and do the push-ups for as long as you can. This is a real challenge, physically and mentally!

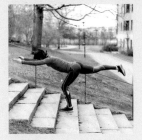

- Warm-up
Pendulum (p. 42)

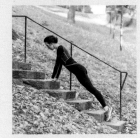

1. Plank (p. 24)

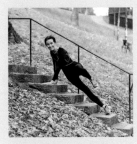

2. Plank 2 (p. 26)

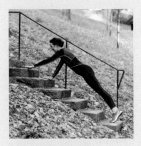

3. Push-ups 3 (p. 39)

HEART RATE CHALLENGE

- **TIME:** 10 minutes
- **EXERCISES:** *Mountain Climbers 1, Burpee, Lunge 2, Mountain Climbers 2*
- **WARM-UP:** *Stair Running*
- **HOW TO:** Warm up with 4 to 5 reps of Stair Running. Set your timer for 10 minutes and perform 5 to 10 exercises, one exercise after the other, in a circuit (but on the stairs). Do as follows: one rep of Mountain Climbers 1, followed by one rep each of Burpees, Lunge 2, and Mountain Climbers 2. When finished, immediately do the set over again. See if you can keep this going for 10 minutes; if not, take small breaks when needed.

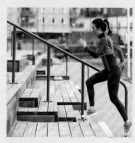

Warm-up
Stair Running (p. 68)

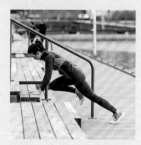

Mountain Climbers 1 (p. 81)

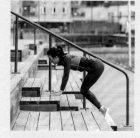

Burpee (p. 72)

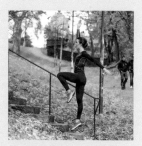

Lunge 2 (p. 22)

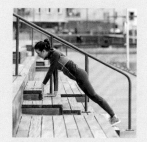

Mountain Climbers 2 (p. 82)

LOWER BODY WORKOUT

- **TIME:** 10 minutes
- **EXERCISES:** *Lunge 3, Stair Jump 1, Lunge 2, Stair Jump 3*
- **WARM-UP:** *Stair Running*
- **HOW TO:** Warm up with 4 to 5 reps of Stair Running. Set your timer for 10 minutes and perform one exercise at a time in a circuit (but on the stairs). Do as follows: One Lunge 3 rep, then a Stair Jump 1, followed by a Lunge 2 and a Stair Jump 3. When done, immediately repeat the set. Try to keep this up for 10 minutes. If you can't, take short breaks when needed.

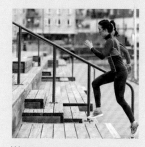

Warm-up
Stair Running (p. 68)

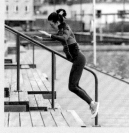

Lunge 3 (p. 23)

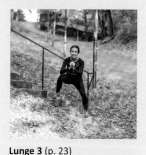

Stair Jump 1 (p. 65)

Lunge 2 (p. 22)

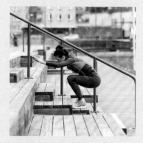

Stair Jump 3 (p. 67)

10-MINUTE FULL-BODY WORKOUT

- **TIME:** 10 minutes
- **EXERCISES:** *Stair Jump 2, Bear Crawl 3, Lunge 2, Push-ups 3*
- **WARM-UP:** *Mountain Climbers 1*
- **HOW TO:** Do 4 reps of a warm-up exercise for 20 seconds per rep to raise your heart rate. Then perform as many repetitions of each exercise as you can manage for two minutes. Finish off by doing another 20-second rep of the warm-up exercise at full speed to use up every remaining ounce of your strength.

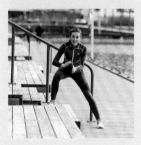

Warm-up
Mountain Climbers 1 (p. 81)

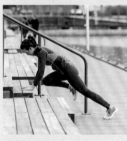

Stair Jump 2 (p. 66)

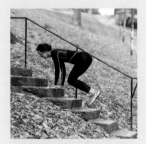

Bear Crawl 3 (p. 35)

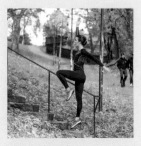

Lunge 2 (p. 22)

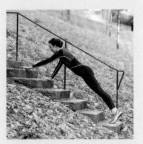

Push-ups 3 (p. 39)

MORE BALANCE

- **TIME:** 15 minutes
- **EXERCISES:** *Pendulum 1, Balance with Leg Lift 3, Handstand, Balance With Step*
- **WARM-UP:** *Pendulum*
- **HOW TO:** Perform the Pendulum as warm-up. Do 5 to 6 reps, or until you feel centered and in tune with your body. Then experiment with the exercises over the quarter hour. Get to know how they feel, see which ones need some fine-tuning, etc. Set this time aside to listen to your body. Focus on what you need right now!

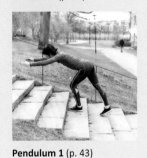

Warm-up
Pendulum (p. 42)

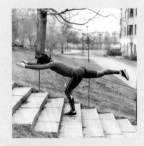

Pendulum 1 (p. 43)

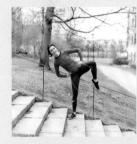

Balance with Leg Lift 3 (p. 53)

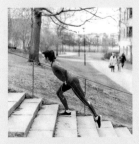

Handstand (p. 46)

Balance with Step 1 (p. 59)

STRENGTH WORKOUT

- **TIME:** 16 minutes
- **EXERCISES:** *Burpee, Push-ups 1, Lunge 1, Lunge 2*
- **WARM-UP:** *Burpee 2* or *Stair Running*
- **HOW TO:** Download the app "Tabata timer" before you begin. Perform your choice of warm-up activity for 1 to 2 minutes. Then do a Tabata-style workout (i.e., 8 reps of each exercise at 20 seconds per rep) before proceeding to the next exercise. This lets you train many parts of your body efficiently in a very short amount of time.

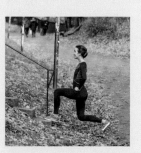 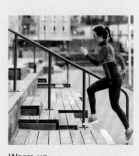

Warm-up
Stair Running (p. 68) alt. **Burpee 2** (p. 74)

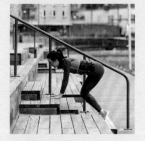

Burpee (p. 72)

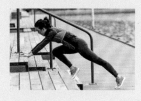

Push-ups 1 (p. 37)

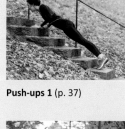

Lunge 1 (p. 21)

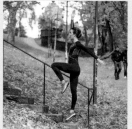

Lunge 2 (p. 22)

RAW STRENGTH 2.0

- **TIME:** 16 minutes
- **EXERCISES:** *Hip Lift 1, Plank 3, Push-ups 3, Bear Crawl 1*
- **WARM-UP:** *Burpee 2*
- **HOW TO:** Download the app "Tabata timer" before you begin. Perform your choice of warm-up activity for 1 to 2 minutes. Then perform the exercises Tabata-style (i.e., 8 reps of each exercise at 20 seconds per rep) before moving on to the next exercise. Hopefully this will lead you to fatigue.

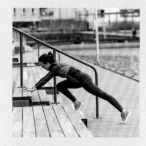

Warm-up
Burpee 2 (p. 74)

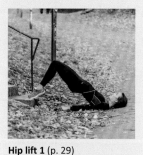 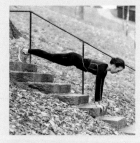

Hip lift 1 (p. 29)

Plank 3 (p. 27)

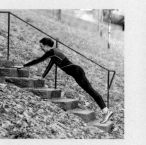 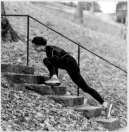

Push-ups 3 (p. 39)

Bear Crawl 1 (p. 33)

IN BALANCE

I'd like to remind you of an essential tenet of health and exercise. I notice that many people forget what should be utterly self-evident: that you must listen to and cooperate with your body. You should take the time to try to decipher and understand your body's signals and respect them. Oftentimes we forget to pay heed to our body and become overwhelmed. We charge full speed ahead, emulate what other people are doing, set the bar far too high, and want to do everything at once. We judge everything we do in such a way that living a healthy lifestyle has become yet one more pursuit in which we are driven to excel.

What compounds the problem is that social media often only shows us what is considered "perfect." We're bombarded on a daily basis with photos of people who seem to live a flawless existence, so it's no surprise that we often forget our humanness and push ourselves to the brink. Some people believe there's too much focus on physical exercise today, and that it has built up to a sort of frenzy. This is true, to certain degree. This so-called training hype is interesting because it concerns mostly individuals who already exercise, and not so much those who still need to find the inspiration to move. People who already work out become more extreme in their training, which can lead to poor health, while those who are not physically active are put off and become even more resistant to exercise, also endangering their health. No matter how we look at this, what's often missing is balance—that midpoint where there's just the right amount of everything.

Personally, I have trouble with the concept that more is always better; too many of us feel obliged to constantly perform and excel. It must be all or nothing all the time, and little is considered satisfactory, or even pleasant, anymore. It's frustrating, and also dangerous, that "good enough" has turned into something subpar and dated. Exercising for its own sake isn't deemed exciting, but boot-camp classes and marathon training are. It's all about raw foods, veganism, being gluten-free, and eating super healthy all the time, all at once. We must be happy, ambitious, successful, good-looking, skilled, and still have a bit of life left in us.

Why must everything be taken to extremes? Why can't health and training be pursuits that make us healthier and stronger, instead of being just another field of high achievement? It makes me sad to see young girls exercise several times a day and live on cottage cheese, thinking that it's healthy. Training several times a day, or every day of the week for that matter, is the domain of elite athletes, not ordinary exercisers with full-time jobs who simply wish to take care of their health.

I wish it were more widely understood that exercise is indeed excellent, but only when it is balanced with sufficient doses of rest. Doing a little but often is better than doing fewer but more strenuous sessions. Exercise should be fun and fill you with energy. It is a gift to yourself. It belongs to you and does not need to be evaluated by anybody else. Training and movement are of equal value, and they should happen on your terms. Training is a break from performance.

In this book, I hope I've proven that exercise can be so simple that you don't need any kind of equipment to engage in it. I want to remind you that it's what you do that counts, and that training shouldn't be a way to measure yourself against others; it should be an activity that brings vigor and joy to your life. I want this book to remind you that training is there for you, if and when you want it. It can be whatever you'd like it to be. You don't have to share your training regimen on Instagram, and you don't need to train every day. You don't even have to scrutinize it if you don't want to—you can train because it makes you feel good. You don't have to perform all the exercises or workouts in this book. You don't always need a strategy; you can choose to tackle whatever makes you feel good today. You can decide to go out and move your body because it makes you feel strong right now. It's not important that you follow the three training programs in this book to the letter, do a hundred burpees, or run several miles. What's important is that you provide your body with regular movement that you enjoy.

OUR WANTS AND NEEDS

I met a very wise person in the fall of 2013, who quickly became a dear friend. Her name is Anna Cederstam-Krantz, and she taught me a fundamental lesson about our wants and needs. Human beings tend to be led by pleasure's strong pull, without any thought to consequences. We want to have fun. We want to give in to what's tempting, and we often pay more heed to that instinct than thinking about what will ensue. This isn't always wrong, but it can occasionally lead us to stop listening to our bodies, which in turn can impede us from making healthy choices.

How often do we really stop and feel and really pay attention to what we need? Today, many people's needs and wants are often strongly disconnected. How many times have you thought to yourself, "But I'm having so much fun, I can sleep on the weekend" or "Sure, my body is completely exhausted, but this workout/social situation/job is so much fun?" I'd like to encourage you to begin asking yourself more often: "What do I want right now?", and then ask yourself the follow-up question: "What do I need right now?" Do you come up with the same reply to those two questions, or are the answers totally different? Which one should you listen to right now?

Here's a simple example: You've worked hard this entire week and have put in many overtime hours at your job. You've crammed your weekend with workouts and social commitments. You think it's going to be great to do something other than work, but on the other hand you feel completely burned out and deep down you'd rather get some rest, physically and mentally. You want to lounge on the couch, go for long walks, and let yourself recover, without having to follow a to-do list. You want to be yourself and allow yourself to be spontaneous. Instead, you stick with your plans and keep your commitments. You do each planned workout, becoming even more fatigued. You attend the dinner parties and by Sunday evening you're completely exhausted. But hey, it was so much fun! Or was it? Here we can see clearly that what you wanted and what you needed were two different things, and that you would have done much better for yourself if you had listened more closely to what you needed.

I think we're so busy "living life"—being seen and heard, being up and about and available—that we neglect what is most important: heeding the messages between our body and our brain. We think logically, but do not feel. We plan without being realistic. We fill in all the time slots with external activities without setting aside some time for ourselves, which should be considered just as vital. Our desire to fit everything in means that we don't have time to communicate with our body. Just look at how we treat our food: Instead of enjoying what is already in our mouth, we gear up for a second bite of cake while we're still chewing on our first forkful.

HEALTH ANALYSIS

One of the most significant things you can do when going over your health and training is to start with an assessment of your needs. You must put together an overall picture of your reality and keep it in mind when you decide to make a change. I always refer back to this health questionnaire

1. **How do you feel right now?**
   Turn off your phone, close your eyes, and really examine how you feel. At this point, you need to be truthful with yourself. How are you, deep down inside? What feelings do you have, or what feelings are coming to the surface?

2. **How does your body feel?**
   Is it alert, sad, off-kilter, or do you feel great? If you truly check, how does your body feel? Do you suffer from any pain? How is your stomach? Do you feel strong? How are things now compared to how you felt a few weeks ago, a few months ago?

3. **Do you like yourself? What do you like? What would you like to change, and why?**
   Provide detailed answers.

4. **When did you last pay yourself a compliment, say a kind word, or have a caring thought?**
   Practice using your thoughts for boosting your self-esteem, instead of putting yourself down. Think a kind thought. Think about what you say to yourself and the reasons behind it.

5. **What is your relationship with your body?**
   Can you compare your relationship to your body to your relationship with a distant cousin, a passionate lover, or a strict parent? What kind of relationship would you like to have with your body? Are there certain parts of your body you like better than others?

6. **How often do you feel stressed out, and in what types of situations? How do you handle stress? At any time, have you felt that the stress was overwhelming?**
   Write down examples and try to find ways to minimize stress in these situations.

7. **Is there anything missing from your health?**
   What do you want for your health, and what can you improve right now that can become part of a long-term plan? Can you set yourself a few kinder, part-time goals and a bigger, long-term goal? Can you start by adding in something healthy from time to time?

8. **Do you exercise as often as you'd like? If not, what gets in your way?**
   Think about how much time you want to devote to your training, and what's realistic for you in your specific situation. Check your schedule and see where it might be possible to add small bouts of exercise. Perhaps you can spare 20 minutes on a Wednesday, or 30 minutes during your lunch break on Fridays. Think short and effective, instead of long and time-consuming.

9. **How often are you sick? Do you notice a pattern?**
   If you always get sick on the first day of a vacation, it might be a sign that you need to reduce your stress at work.

10. **What do you dream of?**
    If you could lead the best, most invigorating lifestyle and be at your healthiest, what would that look like? How far from that point do you find yourself today? Choose three little things that you can try to improve right now. It need not be anything more daring than decreasing your coffee intake, taking a walk for a quarter of an hour each day, or going through your closet to locate the clothes you actually like to wear.

How did it feel to answer these questions? What do you think your answers say about your present health? Is there anything you feel an immediate need to change?

my online courses, and in the advice I give to my clients. Read through the questions on the left-hand page in peace and quiet to give yourself an honest chance to get something out of them. Write down the answers on a piece of paper so that you truly express how you feel. If you can't do it right now, I sincerely hope that you will return to that page again sometime soon.

CREATE SENSIBLE OPTIONS

To reinforce your commitment to training, it's important that you take the opportunity to create sensible options. You need to look at your starting point and take baby steps according to your abilities today. To do this you have to look at a few things, by which I mean you need to ask yourself the following:

1. What are your abilities right now, taking into account your work, everyday life, body, and soul?
2. What can be changed realistically over a short time? They say it takes 21 days to change a habit, so don't start out too forcefully.
3. What can be modified realistically over a longer period of time, say, over a year or two?
4. Do you work with yourself and your body? If not, why not? How can you go about changing this?
5. Do you have a soft starting point, or do you mostly want to change because you've "had enough of being like this" or you "feel like you have to do something?"
6. Do you tend to dwell on what you've already done, or on what you've missed, or on what you didn't have the energy or the time to accomplish?
7. What have you learned from past health challenges, diets, or lifestyle changes? What worked well for you and what do think could be omitted?
8. Can the step training featured in this book help you reach your goals, make you feel better, and get your body to work better? How are you going to make use of this book and its exercises?

ONE LAST THING

In conclusion, I want to remind you that when it comes to training, the most important thing is to not make things complicated—keep it simple so that it works for you. I have written this book with a clear theme to encourage more people to dare to let go of performance anxiety, and to get busy instead. It doesn't always need to involve expensive gym memberships, advanced routines, or many hours of planning ahead. Training can also be impromptu movement, efficient workouts done on stairs, and even play. It can be done without premeditation and be full of pleasure and spontaneity. I encourage you to ignore pressure and status, and just get out there and do . . . something! Maybe today's the day you attempt a handstand against a wall for the very first time, or sprint to the playground with your kids. Perhaps this is the week you don't plan ahead, but simply ask yourself, as you head out for a workout, what you feel like doing today. Maybe today's the day you leave all the equipment at home, lace up your running shoes, and run as far as your legs will take you—or up the stairs—to feel the exhilaration of never getting tired. Run, dear friends, just run!

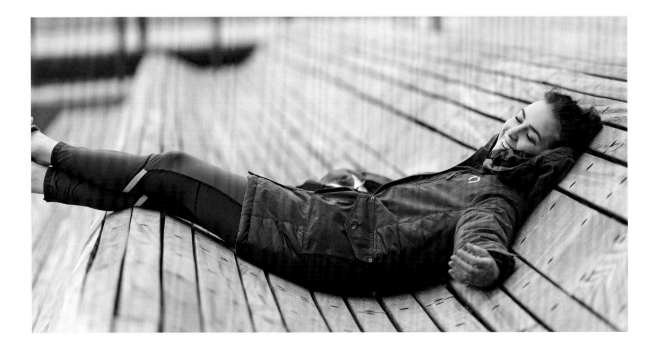

THANK YOU!

I'm incredibly grateful and happy that I was given the opportunity to write this book. It was well worth the effort and time. I'd like to convey sincere thank-yous to the following people:

Kim, because you want to be mine.
My family, because you're always there for me.
My friends, because that's who you are—true friends.

Erik, because you always deliver.
Anders, because you're the best of the best at what you do, every day of the week.
Bonnier Fakta, because you believe in me and you're brilliant to work with.
Cilla, because you're the best and smartest editor.

My blog readers and followers, because you make my work possible. I am forever grateful to you!

Thank you for being a part of my life!

EXERCISE INDEX